DOMINATE

*Optimize your body for
vitality and longevity
In 21 Days with a Vegetarian lifestyle*

BY
MAYA MONDESI

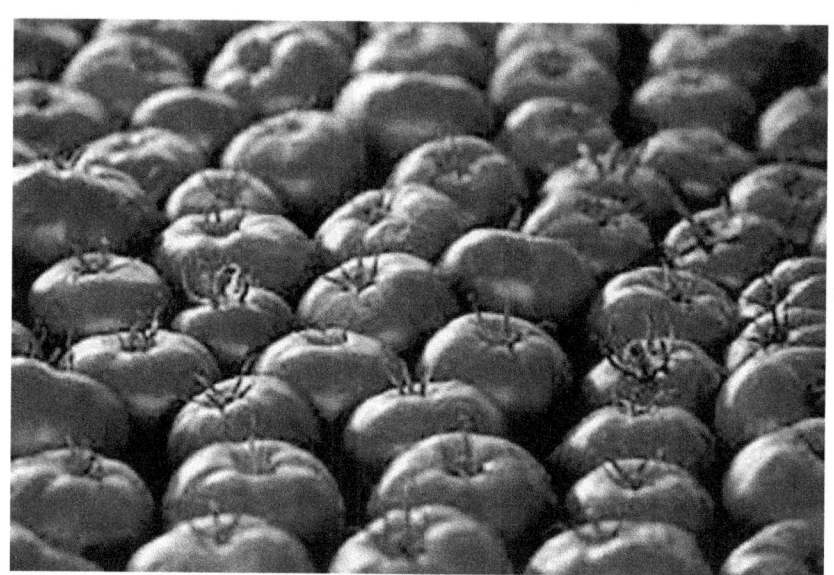

Contents

INTRODUCTION 1
CHAPTER 1: WHAT IS A VEGETARIAN? 2
    Vegetarianism 3
    Who is the Vegetarian Lifestyle Best For? 4
    Ovo-vegetarian 4
CHAPTER 2: THE BASICS OF A VEGETARIAN DIET 5
    I Beat The Reasons for a Vegetarian Diet 6
CHAPTER 3: HOW EXPENSIVE IS A VEGETARIAN DIET? ... 7
    Tips For Cheap Vegetarian Dishes 8
CHAPTER 4: HOW TO BECOME VEGETARIAN 11
    Tips for A Vegetarian Start 11
CHAPTER 5: BENEFITS OF BEING A VEGETARIAN 13
    SAMPLE MENU PLAN 17
CHAPTER 6: BREAKFAST RECIPES 21
    Scrambled Eggs with Cheese 21
    Caramelized Banana Dark Chocolate Oatmeal 23
    Egg Muffins 25
    Chickpea Flour Pancakes 26
    Rhubarb Mango Oatmeal 28
    Easy Tomato Omelets 30
    Mediterranean Breakfast Burrito 32
    Eggs in a Cloud 34
    The 2 Ingredient Banana Egg Pancakes 36
    Coffee Chia Breakfast Pudding 37

Kale, Tomato & Poached Egg on Toast 38

Fried egg Florentine toasties 39

Apple Pie Overnight Oats 41

Banana Peanut Butter Tortilla 43

Apple Carrot Muffin 44

Quinoa & Black Bean Breakfast for Weight Loss 46

Buckwheat Waffles Gluten Free Breakfast 48

Zucchini Muffins 50

CHAPTER 7: LUNCH RECIPES 52

Easy Huevos Rancheros 52

Seasoned Brown Lentils 54

The Runner's Sandwich 56

Hummus and Veggie Roll Ups 58

Coleslaw & Swiss Melt Sandwich 60

Chickpea Salad 62

Glowing Green Hummus 64

Ricotta & White Bean Fancy Toast 66

Perfect Hard-Boiled Eggs (How Long to Boil) 68

Avocado Toast with Egg 70

Sweet Potato Noodles Stir-Fry 72

Ricotta and Spinach Calzones 74

Lentil Tortilla Soup 76

Cold Spicy Peanut Sesame Noodles 78

Spinach, Artichoke and Goat Cheese Quiche 80

Roasted Chickpea Gyros 82

Crispy Baked Black Bean & Sweet Potato Tacos 84

Vegetarian Lettuce Wraps 86

Peanut tofu buddha bowl 88

Harissa Portobello Mushroom "Tacos" 90

CHAPTER 8: DINNER RECIPES **92**

Baked Easy Cheesy Zucchini Casserole 92

Vegan Coconut Curry 94

One Pot Spinach Rice 96

Spicy Corn Chowder 98

Vegetarian Fajita Pasta 100

Farro Salad with Green Olives, Hazelnuts and Raisins 102

Purple Beetroot Pasta 104

Vegetarian Fried Rice 106

Black Bean Veggie Tacos 108

Pineapple Fried Rice 110

Crustless Spinach Cheese Pie 112

Cauliflower Alfredo with Peas 114

Spicy Black Bean Soup 116

Crispy Tortilla Pizza 119

Roasted Chiles Rellenos with Black Beans 121

Vegetarian Enchiladas 125

Mushroom Wellington with Rosemary and Pecans 128

Roasted Cauliflower Enchiladas 131

Black Bean Chili! 133

Cold Sesame Peanut Noodles 135

CHAPTER 9: DESSERT BASED DIET RECIPES 137
    Baked Apple Pie Taquitos with Cinnamon 137
    Baked Apple with Cinnamon Goat Cheese 140
    Carrot Cake Muffins with Coconut Oil and Nutmeg 142
    Chocolate Chunk Banana Nice Cream with Cinnamon 145
    Clementine Upside Down Cupcakes 147
    Mango Sunrise Ice Cream with Coconut-Lime Dust 150
    Baklava Custard Tart 152
    Chocolate, peanut butter & avocado pudding 154
    Orange & rhubarb amaretti pots 156
    Lemon posset with sugared-almond shortbread 158

Sauces Recipe 160
    Vegetarian Pasta Sauce 160
    Mumbo Sauce 162
    Taco Sauce 164
    Creamy Jalapeno Sauce 166
    Roasted Tomato Sauce 168
    Tomato Sauce with Fresh Vegetables and Basil 170
    Sweet Potato Dip 172
    Vegetarian Crock Pot Spaghetti Sauce 174
    Easy Cherry Sauce 176

CHAPTER 10: SNACKS AND SMOOTHIES RECIPES 178
    Tomato Dip with Grilled Bread 178
    Sweet & Spicy Roasted Party Nuts 180
    Roasted Cauliflower 183
    Perfect Roasted Sweet Potatoes 184

Easy Pineapple Mint Popsicles..186

Sweet & Spicy Roasted Party Nuts...187

The Best Guacamole...189

Perfect Roasted Broccoli..191

Garlic Herb White Bean Dip...193

Aji Verde (Spicy Peruvian Green Sauce) 195

Honey Butter Cornbread...197

Easy Pineapple Mint Popsicles..200

Easy Green Goddess Dressing...201

Smoothie Vegetarian **203**

Strawberry green goddess smoothie...203

Green smoothie...204

Avocado smoothie..206

Carrot and orange smoothie...207

Sunshine smoothie...208

Kale smoothie...209

INTRODUCTION

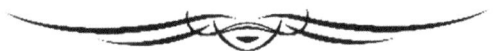

Dominate your health by eating clean. A human body is like a working machine. In order for it to work well it needs to be fueled in the right manner. Nothing will increase people's health and the chance of survival on earth like the step towards a vegetarian diet. The vegetarian way of life is basically suitable for every situation and age.

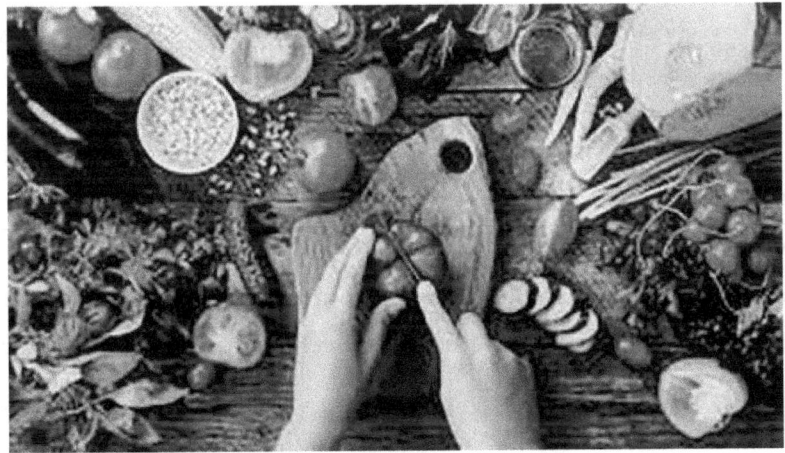

Chapter 1
WHAT IS A VEGETARIAN?

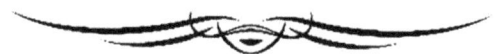

A vegetarian is someone who does not eat meat or fish or other animal products, especially for moral, religious, or health reasons.

Vegetarians do not eat slaughterhouse products or by-products. They do not eat any food that has been prepared using technological aids for slaughter. Vegetable meats don't taste the same as animal meats, but many people like them more.

A vegetarian lifestyle is one in which the person doing it is aware of the origins of the products they use and the food they eat.

Vegetarians do not want to support anything that could cause harm or suffering to animals. Therefore, strict definitions have at most one function: to provide an overview. No vegetarian definition can adequately express the plant philosophy of life with its individual characteristics. Vegetarian beginners, therefore, should not stop at the definitions, but start where they think is correct.

Vegetarianism

Many people are inaccurate about vegetarianism and what it might represent. Vegetarianism is the act of ousting the use of meat (red meat, poultry, fish and the substance of some other creature) and can also incorporate the abstention from the side effects of the creature's butcher.

Vegetarianism could be embraced for several reasons. There are numerous individual articles and documentries on meat consumption keeping in mind conscious life. These moral inspirations have been systematized under different rigorous beliefs, just like the support of basic human rights. Various inspirations for vegetarianism are related to well-being, political, ecological, social, fashionable, financial, or individual inclination. There are also varieties of the food routines: a diet for ovo-lactose vegetable lovers incorporates the two eggs and dairy products, an ovo-vegetarian diet incorporates eggs, but not dairy products, and a lactose-vegetarian diet incorporates dairy products but not eggs. A demanding vegetarian diet excludes every single creature object, including eggs and dairy products. The shirking of creature objects may require dietary improvements to avoid deficiencies; for example, the nutritional insufficiency of B12. Psychologically, the inclination for nourishment for vegetable lovers can be influenced by their financial status and variables of development.

Who is the Vegetarian Lifestyle Best For?

Like many, vegetable lovers may count calories also. However, the purposes behind a diet for most vegetable lovers is not for weightloss purposes but usually for medical benefits; such as to reduce the risk of coronary heart disease, diabetes, and some malignancies.

Some vegetarians depend too intensely on managed nutrients, which can be high in calories, sugar, fat, and sodium. In addition, they may not eat enough natural products, vegetables, whole grains, and calcium-rich foods, subsequently transferring the supplements they give.

In any case, with a touch of organization of a vegetable-loving diet that can address the issues of people all things considered, including children, young people, and pregnant women or the sick. The key is to know your nutritional needs in order to plan a food routine that will satisfy them.

Ovo-vegetarian

People who don't eat meat or dairy products but eat eggs can be referred to as egg-vegetarians. Many follow this diet plan simply because they are lactose intolerant, making digestion of most dairy products difficult.

Chapter 2
THE BASICS OF A VEGETARIAN DIET

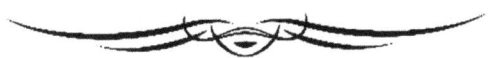

Vegetarian diets are commonly defined by what they exclude rather than what they include. For example, many people refuse to allow eggs on a vegetarian diet, while others, particularly in the UK, also prohibit certain types of cheese on a vegetarian diet, probably due to the use of rennet, which is of animal origin. In the 1960s and 1970s, when vegetarianism began to spread in the United States, so-called homemade salad and pasta dishes were often the only options available for vegetarians on restaurant menus. But as awareness grew and adoption spread in the 1980s, 1990s, and the 21st century, the rich variety of a vegetarian diet gained commercial appeal. Restaurant kitchens from fast food to fine dining now offer tasty and imaginative vegetarian dishes that appeal to both meat and non-meat eaters.

A vegetarian diet includes plenty of fruit and vegetables, beans and legumes, whole and ancient cereals such as rice, wheat, barley, millet, teff, oats, quinoa, buckwheat and amaranth, soy products such as edamame and tofu, meat substitutes such as vegetarian burgers, vegetarian "chicken," tempeh and seitan, baked goods and bread including biscuits, cakes, croissants and bagels, nuts and seeds, including non-dairy milk such as almonds, hemp and flax; all varieties of wheat and non-wheat pasta, algae such as nori and wakame, oils, condiments including herbs and spices, and spicy sauce, soy sauce and nama shoyu. Lacto-ovo vegetarians also eat eggs and egg products, as well as dairy products such as ice cream, cheese, milk, cream, and butter. Some global cuisines, such as Indian, Ethiopian, and Burmese, rely heavily on plant-based meals, but other meat-loving cultures produce some of the most inventive vegetarian dishes, such as Chinese, Mexican, and Italian.

I Beat The Reasons for a Vegetarian Diet

People can choose a vegetarian diet for simple preference, for ethical or religious beliefs, or for its widely recognized health benefits, such as reducing the risk of heart disease and type 2 diabetes. A vegetarian diet can also make it easier to deal with other dietary concerns, such as lactose or gluten intolerance and some food allergies. Plant-based diets have also been proposed as a solution to climate change and can result in lower food expenditure, particularly for those who grow vegetables and herbs in a home garden.

Chapter 3
How Expensive Is a Vegetarian Diet?

The vegetarian diet is suitable for all budgets, and the price of food depends on its level of processing or its quality. The more a food is processed, the more expensive the purchase price in the store. This means that processed foods and convenience products are significantly more expensive than the basic ingredients from which the meal is prepared.

Due to the global network, the discharge of wages abroad, and the different climatic zones, it is possible to obtain fruits and vegetables that would also grow in Europe more economically from distant regions. If you, as a buyer in the supermarket, pay attention to seals such as organic, fair trade, or regional products, you will quickly notice that these products are more expensive. But they are healthy, guarantee a fair distribution of profits, and keep our diet plans.

Think about it. At three or four or more dollars per pound, meat is one of the most expensive items in the grocery store. There are also usually some wastes associated with this. Replacing pounds for pounds with beans (just a simple example, but not too different from what many new vegetarians do) would result in significant savings, as even organic beans cooked in a can can only cost about a dollar per pound. Replacing the meat with tempeh or tofu would be more expensive than replacing it with beans, but this would still not lead to a higher food bill than if you purchased meat.

But that's not really the point. Most vegetarians are not satisfied with simply replacing meat with beans. As you know, you inevitably would want to branch out and explore new foods, which is one of the really great things that happen when you become a vegetarian. As you start eating better, you want to try all the exotic superfoods you learn about to see how incredible food can make you feel.

Tips For Cheap Vegetarian Dishes

Vegetarian nutrition does not need exotic powders and distant berries. This is how you eat a healthy and cheap veggie diet.

» **Don't (always) shop at Whole Foods.**

I know, it's fun. It's Christmas for us veggie food nerds, and there's something to be said for enjoying your shopping experience. But it's also really, really expensive.

Instead, shop at a "normal" grocery store. Many of them now have organic store brands, like Nature's Promise, that cost only slightly more than the non-organic store-brand products.

» **Don't buy everything organic.**

One of the great things about going vegetarian once you are no longer paying for meat, you can invest in the organic stuff that prehaps you could not before. Organic can become addictive, so be careful not to overspend.

The general formula: In a single, large pot, cook the grain of your choice (quinoa and rice) in water with a little salt. Once it's almost done, add the chopped green of your choice (spinach and collards are fun, kale is tough but packed with nutrients). And while that wilts, add the cooked bean or legume of your choice. Then dress it up with sea salt, hot sauce, salsa, vinegar, soy sauce, or whatever else you're in the mood for.

» **Grow your own herbs.**

This tip alone can save you hundreds of dollars per year. For a single bunch of herbs, you'll pay close to what it costs for an already-started plant that you can put on your windowsill or porch and harvest again and again as needed.

» **Make everything you can.**

As busy as we all are now, there's something to be said for paying for convenience. But there's something less obvious to be said for slowing down and spending a couple of hours on a Sunday prepping food for the week, with some music or your spouse or your kid. It's therapeutic.

So instead of buying pre-packaged salad, buy a few heads of greens and chop them yourself. Same with whatever other vegetables you want in there. (A salad spinner is a huge help here.)

And finally, don't forget that you can make your own homemade sports drinks and gels that are far better than most of what's in the stores and cheaper than anything of comparable quality.

» **Don't be afraid to substitute.**

When a recipe calls for chia seeds or toasted sesame oil or tamari, by all means leave it out if you don't already have it! Listen, I know it's fun to make authentic recipes and do them right, but if it's going to make the difference between your going vegetarian and not, skip the fancy stuff at first. Especially when it's something you'll have to buy a whole bottle or jar of and you won't use it again any time soon.

Chapter 4
How to Become Vegetarian

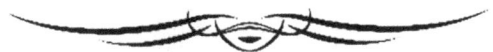

While being a vegetarian isn't for everyone, I talk to lots of people every day who tell me they'd like to become vegetarian but it seems like it would be too hard and they don't have the willpower.

Becoming a vegetarian, for me and for many others, is the easiest thing in the world.

Tips for A Vegetarian Start

» **Cut the fat.**

Which means that by cutting out meat, you'll be cutting out a lot of bad fat, and replacing it with things that are probably not only lower in fat, but more satiating.

» **Less food poisoning.**

Cut out meat and you lower your risk of food poisoning.

» **Reduce the suffering.**

Suffice it to say, there is lots of suffering involved, and by cutting out meat, you are reducing your involvement in that.

- **Help the environment.**

There are actually numerous ways that the meat industry harms the environment, from waste of our resources (animals raised for food eat enough grain to feed the world) to climate change.

- **Help your weight loss.**

If you're trying to lose weight, being a vegetarian can be a good part of your program.

- **Get more nutrition.**

In general (although not necessarily), vegetarians replace meat with more nutritious foods, such as fruits, vegetables, beans, whole grains, and so on.

- **Have good reasons.**

If you just want to become vegetarian for kicks, you probably won't stick with it for long — not because it's hard, but because any lifestyle change or habit change requires a little bit of motivation and discipline.

Chapter 5
BENEFITS OF BEING A VEGETARIAN

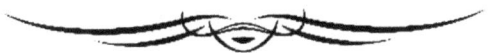

H ealth is the greatest good. Your food is your medicine and your medicine is your food, illness and well-being are directly related to our nutrition.

A plant-based diet has a positive effect on health. A wholesome plant-based diet can help prevent most of the diseases of civilization. Several studies have already shown that a plant-based diet prevents osteoporosis, lowers the risk of type 2 diabetes, protects against high blood pressure, prevents obesity, and serves as prevention against kidney and heart diseases.

» **You'll ward off disease.**

Vegan diets consume fewer calories and are more restorative than the normal American eating routine, especially in forestalling or turning around coronary illness and decreasing the danger of malignant growth. A low-fat veggie lover diet is the absolute best approach to stop the movement of the coronary supply route malady or forestall it totally. Cardiovascular malady slaughters 1 million Americans yearly and is the main source of death in the United States.

> **You'll keep your weight down.**

The standard diet—high in saturated fats and processed foods and low in plant-based foods and complex carbohydrates—is making us fat and killing us slowly.

> **You'll live longer.**

If you switch from the standard American diet to a vegetarian diet, you can add about 13 healthy years to your life. People who consume saturated, four-legged fat have a shorter lifespan and more disability at the end of their lives. Animal products clog your arteries, zap your energy and slow down your immune system. Meat eaters also experience accelerated cognitive and sexual dysfunction at a younger age.

> **You'll build strong bones.**

When there isn't sufficient calcium in the circulation system, our bodies will drain it from existing bone. The metabolic outcome is that our skeletons will get permeable and lose quality after some time. Most insurance experts suggest that we increase our calcium absorpotion using the manner nature planned—through nourishment. Nourish yourself also with different supplements; for example, phosphorus, magnesium, and vitamin D, which are fundamental for the body to assimilate and utilize calcium.

Individuals who are gently lactose-prejudiced can frequently appreciate modest quantities of dairy items; for example, yogurt, cheddar cheese and lactose-free milk. In any case, in the event that you maintain a strategic distance from dairy inside and out, you can get enough calcium from dry beans, tofu, soymilk, and leafy green vegetables; for example, broccoli, kale, collards, and turnip greens.

» **You'll reduce your risk of food-borne illnesses.**

The CDC reports that food-borne illnesses of all kinds account for 76 million illnesses a year, resulting in 325,000 hospitalizations and 5,000 deaths in the United States. According to the US Food and Drug Administration (FDA), foods rich in protein, such as meat, poultry, fish and seafood, are frequently involved in food-borne illness outbreaks.

» **You'll ease the symptoms of menopause.**

Many foods contain nutrients beneficial to perimenopausal and menopausal women. Certain foods are rich in phytoestrogens, the plant-based chemical compounds that mimic the behavior of estrogen. Since phytoestrogens can increase and decrease estrogen and progesterone levels, maintaining a balance of them in your diet helps ensure a more comfortable passage through menopause. Soy is by far the most abundant natural source of phytoestrogens, but these compounds also can be found in hundreds of other foods, such as apples, beets, cherries, dates, garlic, olives, plums, raspberries, squash, and yams. Because menopause is also associated with weight gain and a slowed metabolism, a low-fat, high-fiber vegetarian diet can help ward off extra pounds.

» **You'll have more energy.**

Good nutrition generates more usable energy—energy to keep pace with the kids, tackle that home improvement project, or have better sex more often, Michael F. Roizen, MD, says in The RealAge Diet. Too much fat in your bloodstream means that arteries won't open properly and that your muscles won't get enough oxygen.

» **You'll be more "regular."**

Eating a lot of vegetables necessarily means consuming more fiber, which pushes waste out of the body. Meat contains no fiber. People who eat lower on the food chain tend to have fewer instances of constipation, hemorrhoids, and diverticulitis.

» **You'll help reduce pollution.**

Some people become vegetarians after realizing the devastation that the meat industry is having on the environment. According to the US Environmental Protection Agency (EPA), chemical and animal waste runoff from factory farms is responsible for more than 173,000 miles of polluted rivers and streams. Runoff from farmlands is one of the greatest threats to water quality today. Agricultural activities that cause pollution include confined animal facilities, plowing, pesticide spraying, irrigation, fertilizing and harvesting.

» **Your dinner plate will be full of color.**

Disease-fighting phytochemicals give fruits and vegetables their rich, varied hues. They come in two main classes: carotenoids and anthocyanins. All rich yellow and orange fruits and vegetables—carrots, oranges, sweet potatoes, mangoes, pumpkins, corn—owe their color to carotenoids. Leafy green vegetables also are rich in carotenoids but get their green color from chlorophyll. Red, blue, and purple fruits and vegetables—plums, cherries, red bell peppers—contain anthocyanins. Cooking by color is a good way to ensure you're eating a variety of naturally occurring substances that boost immunity and prevent a range of illnesses.

SAMPLE MENU PLAN

	BREKFAST	LUNCH	DINNER	SNACKS/ SMOOTHIES	DESSERT/ SAUCES
S	Scrambled Eggs with Cheese	Seasoned Brown Lentils	Baked Easy Cheesy Zucchini Casserole	Sweet & Spicy Roasted Party Nuts	Baked Apple Pie Taquitos with Cinnamon
M	Caramelized Banana Dark Chocolate Oatmeal	Hummus and Veggie Roll Ups	Vegan Coconut Curry	Roasted Cauliflower	Baked Apple with Cinnamon Goat Cheese
T	Egg Muffins	Coleslaw & Swiss Melt Sandwich	One Pot Spinach Rice	Perfect Roasted Sweet Potatoes	Carrot Cake Muffins with Coconut Oil and Nutmeg
W	Chickpea Flour Pancakes	Avocado Toast with Egg	Spicy Corn Chowder	Easy Pineapple Mint Popsicles	Chocolate Chunk Banana Nice Cream with Cinnamon
T	Rhubarb Mango Oatmeal	Chickpea Salad/ The Runner's Sandwich	Vegetarian Fajita Pasta	Sweet & Spicy Roasted Party Nuts/ Tomato Dip with Grilled Bread	Vegetarian Pasta Sauce

DOMINATE

	BREKFAST	LUNCH	DINNER	SNACKS/ SMOOTHIES	DESSERT/ SAUCES
F	Easy Tomato Omelets	Glowing Green Hummus	Farro Salad with Green Olives, Hazelnuts and Raisins	The Best Guacamole	Mumbo Sauce
S	Mediterranean Breakfast Burrito	Ricotta & White Bean Fancy Toast	Purple Beetroot Pasta	Aji Verde	Taco Sauce
S	Scrambled Eggs with Cheese	Perfect Hard-Boiled Eggs (How Long to Boil)	Vegetarian Fried Rice	Honey Butter Cornbread/ Garlic Herb White Bean Dip	Clementine Upside Down Cupcakes
M	Eggs in a Cloud	Coleslaw & Swiss Melt Sandwich	Black Bean Veggie Tacos	Easy Pineapple Mint Popsicles	Mango Sunrise Ice Cream with Coconut-Lime Dust
T	The 2 Ingredient Banana Egg Pancakes	Avocado Toast with Egg	Pineapple Fried Rice	Easy Green Goddess Dressing	Baklava Custard Tart
W	Coffee Chia Breakfast Pudding	Sweet Potato Noodles Stir-Fry	Crustless Spinach Cheese Pie	Strawberry green goddess smoothie	Chocolate, Peanut Butter & Avocado
T	Scrambled Eggs with Cheese	Ricotta and Spinach Calzones	Cauliflower Alfredo with Peas	Green smoothie	Creamy Jalapeno Sauce

{18}

BENEFITS OF BEING A VEGETARIAN

	BREKFAST	LUNCH	DINNER	SNACKS/SMOOTHIES	DESSERT/SAUCES
F	Kale, tomato & poached egg on toast	Lentil Tortilla Soup	Spicy Black Bean Soup	Avocado smoothie	Roasted Tomato Sauce
S	Fried egg Florentine toasties	Cold Spicy Peanut Sesame Noodles	Crispy Tortilla Pizza	Carrot and Orange Smoothie	Tomato Sauce with Fresh Vegetables and Basil
S	Apple Pie Overnight Oats	Spinach, Artichoke and Goat Cheese Quiche	Crispy Tortilla Pizza	Easy Pineapple Mint Popsicles	Chocolate Chunk Banana Nice Cream
M	Banana Peanut Butter Tortilla	Roasted Chickpea Gyros	Roasted Chiles Rellenos with Black Beans	Perfect Roasted Sweet Potatoes	Creamy Jalapeno Sauce
T	Apple Carrot Muffin	Crispy Baked Black Bean & Sweet Potato Tacos	Vegetarian Enchiladas	Guacamole	Baked Apple with Cinnamon Goat Cheese
W	Quinoa & Black Bean Breakfast for Weight Loss	Vegetarian Lettuce Wraps/ Easy Huevos Rancheros	Mushroom Wellington with Rosemary and Pecans	Sunshine smoothie	Orange & Rhubarb Amaretti Pots

T	Buckwheat Waffles Gluten Free Breakfast	Peanut Tofu Buddha Bowl	Roasted Cauliflower Enchiladas	Cornbread	Mumbo Sauce
F	Zucchini Muffins	Harissa Portobello Mushroom "Tacos"	Black Bean Chili	Easy Pineapple Mint Popsicles	Lemon Posset with Sugared-Almond Shortbread
S	Scrambled Eggs with Cheese	Coleslaw & Swiss Melt Sandwich	Cold Sesame Peanut Noodles	Kale smoothie	Chocolate, Peanut Butter & Avocado

Chapter 6

Breakfast Recipes

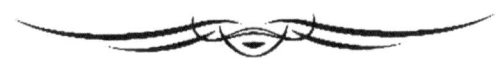

Scrambled Eggs with Cheese

Prep Time:2 mins - Cook Time:3 mins - Total Time:5 mins

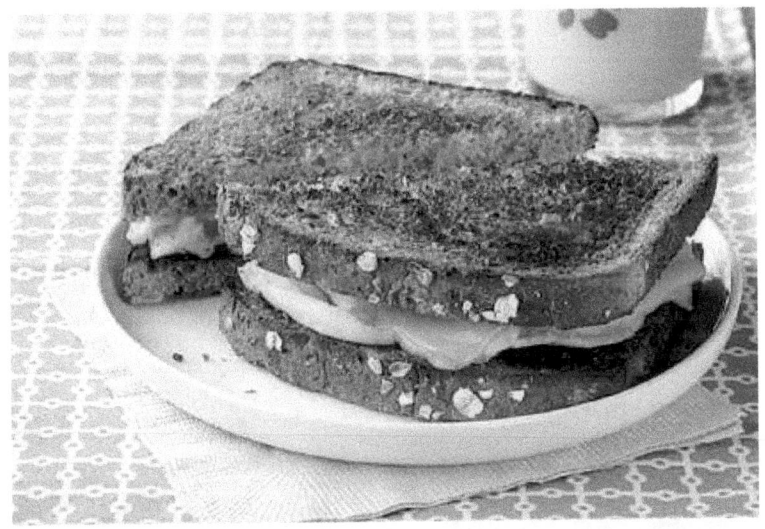

Ingredients

- 2 eggs
- ½ cup cheddar cheese, grated (or Monterey Jack)
- 1 tbsp butter (or olive oil)
- salt and pepper to taste
- Optional:
- 1 slice whole grain toast

Preparation

- Put a pan onto a medium heat and put in the butter or oil.
- Break the eggs into a bowl and beat quickly with a fork.
- Add some salt and pepper to the egg mix.
- Grate the cheese and have it ready.
- Tip the beaten eggs into the frying pan.
- Layer the cheese on top.
- The eggs will start to solidify almost straight away - as soon as they do use a spatula and 'pull' the eggs in from the side to the middle.
- Repeat the pulling in several times.
- It doesn't take long, the idea behind this is you'll have soft, lightly cooked fresh eggs. It's hard to undercook an egg really, but very easy to overcook. 2 - 3 mins cooking time is all you'll need.
- When the egg has no 'watery' bits left, you're done! Quickly remove from heat and transfer to plate - preferably on top of some lovely, hot, unbuttered toast.

BREAKFAST RECIPES

Caramelized Banana Dark Chocolate Oatmeal

Cook Time: 10 min - Total Time: 10 mins

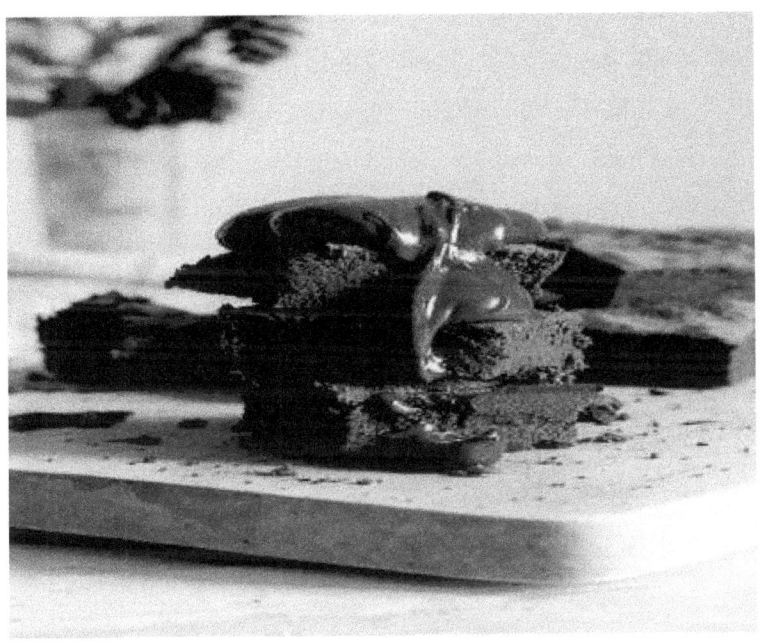

Ingredients

- » 1 cup water
- » 1/2 cup rolled oats
- » Olive oil spray
- » 1/2 medium banana, sliced
- » 1 tbsp dark chocolate chips*

Preparation

- In a small saucepan, bring water to a boil. Stir in oats and reduce heat to low. Simmer until oats have absorbed all of the liquid, 3-5 mins.
- While oats are cooking, spray a small non-stick skillet with olive oil. Add sliced bananas in a single layer and cook over medium heat until caramelized, about 3 mins per side.
- Spoon oatmeal into a bowl and top with caramelized bananas, and chocolate chips.

Egg Muffins

Prep: 15 Mins - Cook: 20 Mins - Total: 35 Mins

Ingredients

- 1 bell pepper, red
- 2 spring onions
- 6 eggs
- 1 handful spinach (or any green leaves)
- ½ cup cheddar cheese (grated; other cheese is fine too)
- 1 tsp salt
- 4-5 splashes hot sauce (or 1 tsp curry powder)

Preparation

- Preheat the oven to 200°C/ 390°F.
- Wash and dice the bell pepper and onions. and put them in a large mixing bowl.
- Wash the spinach, lightly chop it and add it to the bowl as well.
- Add the eggs and salt. Mix well. Pro tip – crack the eggs separately before adding. That way if you get a dodgy one, it won't ruin the whole meal.
- Mix in the cheese to the batter.
- Add some hot sauce or curry powder.
- Grease the muffin tin with oil and kitchen paper/baking brush and pour the egg mixture evenly into the muffin slots. (If you think they might still stick to the pan use some muffin cups or cut out some baking paper and to use as cups – definitely saves time on doing the washing up
- Pop the tray into the oven for 20 mins or until the tops are firm to the touch.

Chickpea Flour Pancakes

Prep Time 5 mins - Cook Time 5 mins - Total Time 10 mins

Ingredients

- 1 cup chickpea flour (or bean/garbanzo flour)
- 1 cup water
- 1 tsp turmeric
- ½ tsp salt
- ½ tsp pepper
- 3 spring onions
- 1 tbsp olive oil (ghee would be perfect here, but not vegan)
- Optional
- ½ tsp chili flakes (I highly recommend this)
- 1 bell pepper, red
- ½ cup peas

Preparation

- Add the flour, water, turmeric, salt, pepper and chili flakes (if using) to a mixing bowl and give it a quick blend using a food processor or blender. Leave it to settle for a few mins while you heat up the oil or ghee in a non-stick pan. The batter needs to look very runny!
- Dice the veggies finely and add them to the mixture.
- Use a tissue or similar (a spray oil would work wonders here) to ensure the bottom of the pan is coated well in oil.
- Add about a ladle of the mixture and veggies when the pan is hot - a medium heat should be just right.

- Cook for about 3 mins - the mixture will quickly start to firm. If you're using two pans, you can make two pancakes at the same time.
- Make sure you use a large pan (or pans) here, you're aiming for thin pancakes. They're MUCH easier to handle!
- Use a large spatula to help you flip the pancakes, adding more oil underneath if necessary. After another 2-3 mins your pancake will be ready!
- Keep it somewhere warm while you repeat with the second pancake, adding more oil when necessary.
- Done! Add your desired toppings and enjoy. Remember - it's important to eat these pancakes warm - don't let them get cold!

Rhubarb Mango Oatmeal

Prep Time 5 mins - Cook Time 10 mins - Total Time 15 mins

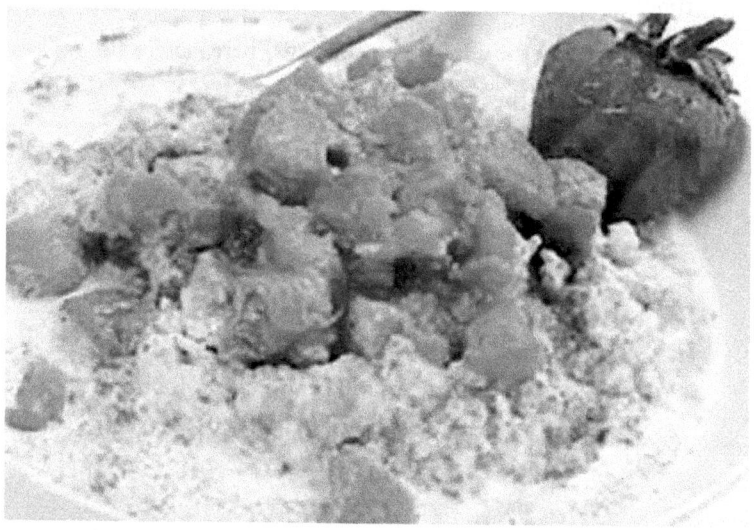

Ingredients

- 1/2 cup chopped rhubarb
- 1 pitted date or dash of sweetener of your choice
- 1/2 cup almond milk more if necessary
- 1/3 cup rolled oats
- 1/2 cup diced mango frozen or fresh
- 1 tsp lemon zest more if you love zest!
- 1 tsp chia seeds
- dash salt

Preparation

- Place rhubarb and date in a saucepan.
- Add a quarter cup water to the pan and simmer until rhubarb softens. 3-4 mins
- Add almond milk and turn up the heat to medium high until the mixture is just about to boil.
- Reduce the heat and add oats. Cook 3 mins until oats are almost done.
- Add mango, lemon zest, chia and dash of salt. Stir to combine.
- Simmer until heated through and oats are done (especially if using frozen mango).

Easy Tomato Omelets

Prep Time: 2 mins - Cook Time: 8 mins - Total Time: 10 minS

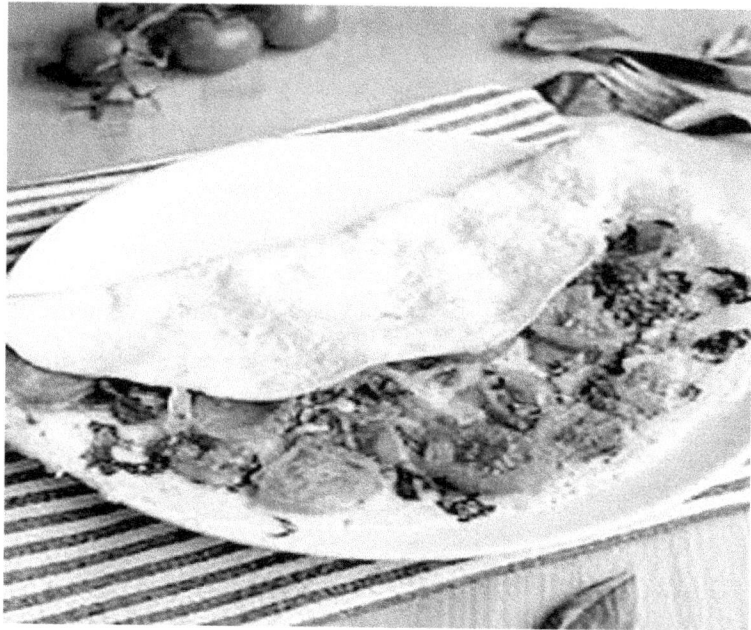

Ingredients

- 2 eggs
- 2 tbsp olive oil
- ½ cup cherry tomatoes (the sweeter the better)
- ½ cup basil, fresh (dried will work if necessary)
- ¼ cup favourite cheese (think cheddar, monterey jack, mozzarella, remember to avoid rennet if you're vegetarian)
- salt and pepper to taste
- Optional:
- 2 spring onions
- 1 chili (red or green)

Preparation

- Wash the tomatoes (and spring onions or chili if you're using them) and chop into small pieces.
- Heat oil in a pan and fry the tomatoes for about 2 mins. Set aside. Clean the pan with a tissue.
- Crack the eggs into a bowl and beat well with a fork, adding the salt and pepper
- Heat the rest of the oil in a pan (non-stick if possible) on low to medium heat
- Pour the egg mix into the pan
- Using a spatula, ruffle the omelette so it doesn't stick. As you create gaps tilt the pan so the liquid fills the spaces.
- Let it cook for about 2 mins and...
- Here's the important part: when the egg mixture looks nearly cooked (but there's still just a tiny bit of runny egg left) drop on the tomatoes and basil (and cheese, spring onions or chili if you're using them).
- Fold the empty half of the omelette on top of the other.
- Slide it onto a plate - the heat from closing the omelette will finish cooking the inside

Mediterranean Breakfast Burrito

Prep Time: 15 mins - Cook Time 5 mins - Total Time 20 mins

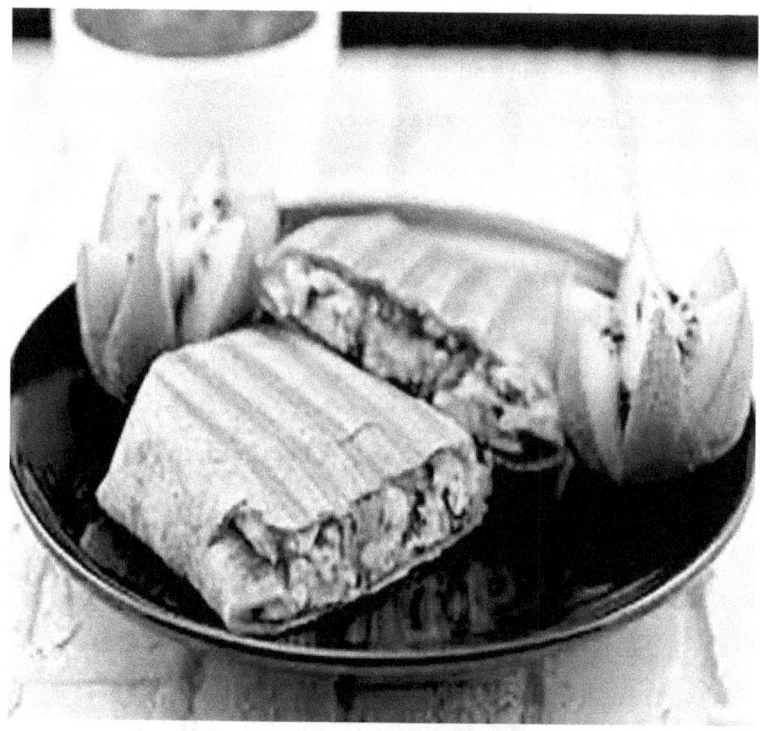

Ingredients

- 6 tortillas whole 10 inch - I use sun-dried tomato
- 9 eggs whole
- 2 cups baby spinach washed and dried
- 3 tbsp black olives sliced
- 3 tbsp sun-dried tomatoes chopped
- 1/2 cup feta cheese I use light/low-fat feta
- 3/4 cup refried beans canned
- Garnish: salsa (optional)

Preparation

- Spray medium frying pan with non- stick spray. Scramble eggs and toss for about 5 mins, or until eggs are no longer liquid. Add spinach, black olives, sun-dried tomatoes and continue to stir/toss until no longer wet. Add feta cheese and cover until cheese is melted.
- Add 2 tbsp of refried beans to each tortilla. Top with egg mixture, dividing evenly between all burritos. Wrap as shown in video.
- Grill on panini press (this is what I use) or in frying pan until lightly browned.
- Serve hot with salsa and fruit (optional)
- If freezing: wait until cooled, then wrap as directed in video.
- If you are reheating: Heat in microwave (in parchment paper) for about 2 mins. Serve hot.

DOMINATE

Eggs in a Cloud

Total: 20 min - Active: 10 min

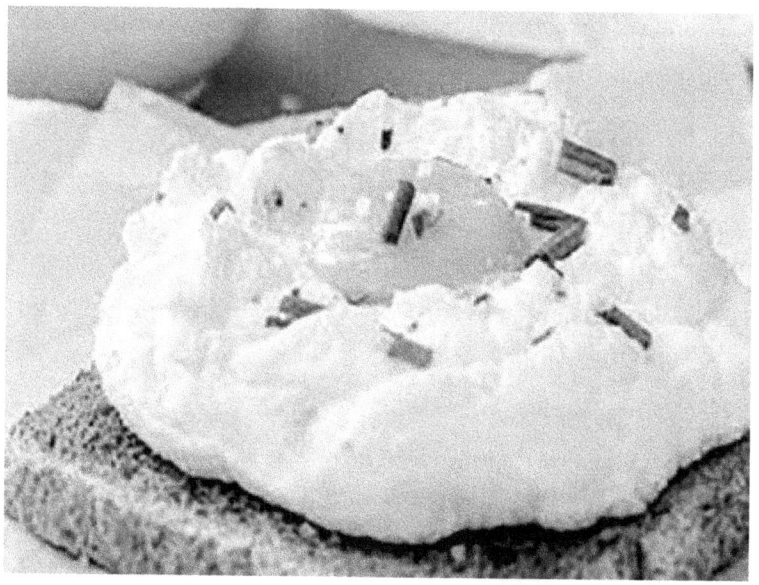

Ingredients

- » 4 large free-range eggs
- » 2 tbsp chives finely chopped
- » 3 rashers Quorn vegetarian bacon finely chopped
- » a generous pinch of sea salt
- » freshly cracked black pepper to taste

Preparation

- Preheat oven to 220C / 450F, and line a baking tray with parchment paper.
- Carefully separate the egg whites from the yolk, making sure not to break the yolks.
- Add the egg whites and a pinch of salt in a stand mixer with a whisk attachment, and whisk the egg whites until stiff peaks form. Gently mix in the chives and bacon bits.
- Spoon the egg whites mixture into even little clouds over your prepared baking tray.
- Arrange the baking tray the middle rack of your oven, and bake the egg whites for 3 mins.
- Gently place 1 egg yolk on top of each cloud, and bake for a further 3 mins.
- Remove from the oven and serve immediately, with freshly cracked black pepper on top.

The 2 Ingredient Banana Egg Pancakes

Prep Time: 5 Mins To 10 Mins - Cook Time: 2 Mins To 3 Mins

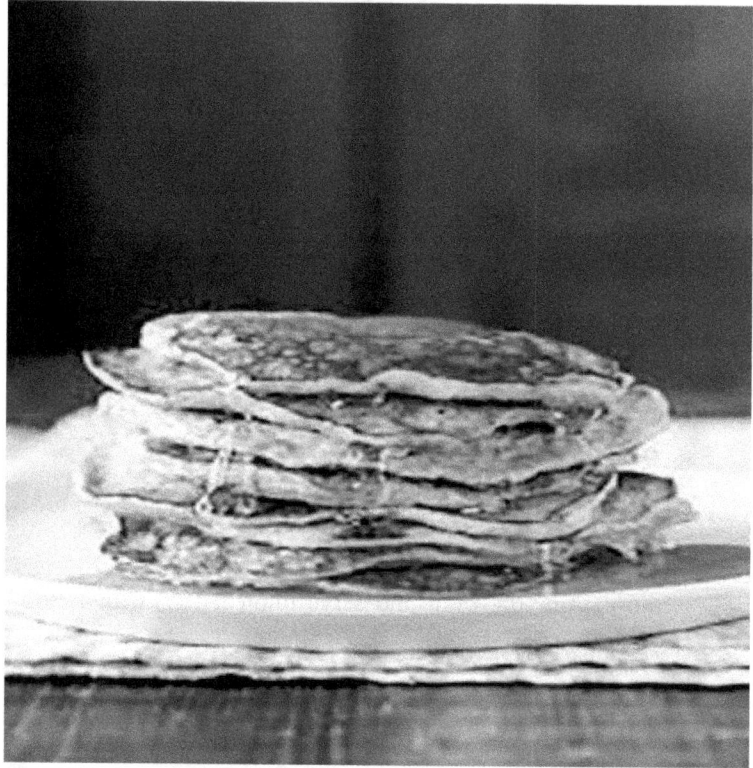

Ingredients

- 1 banana
- 2 eggs

Preparation

- Mash up bananas in a large bowl.
- Whisk eggs (using a fork is just fine!) and add to banana paste.
- Fry gently in a pan on low-medium heat with a little heated oil or butter

Coffee Chia Breakfast Pudding

Prep Time: 3 mins - Total Time: 3 mins

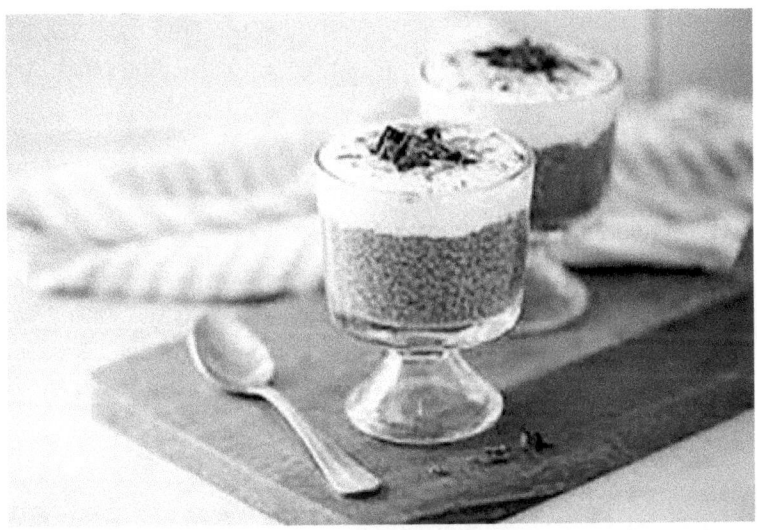

Ingredients

- » 4 heaped tablespoons chia seeds
- » 175 ml coffee freshly brewed and reasonably cooled
- » 175 ml coconut milk full fat, out of a tin - not the low-fat version you buy in a tetra Pak!
- » 1 tbsp almond butter Optional
- » 1 tsp vanilla paste
- » 2 tbsp erythritol
- » 1/2 tsp cinnamon

Preparation

- » Put all ingredients in a bowl and stir.
- » Cover and refrigerate overnight.

Kale, Tomato & Poached Egg on Toast

Prep: 2 Mins - Cook: 7 Min

Ingredients

- 2 tsp oil
- 100g ready-chopped kale
- 1 garlic clove, crushed
- ½ tsp chilli flakes
- 2 large eggs
- 2 slices multigrain bread
- 50g cherry tomatoes, halved
- 15g feta, crumbled

Preparation

- Bring a large pan of water to the boil. Heat the oil in a frying pan over a medium heat and add the kale, garlic and chilli flakes. Cook, stirring occasionally, for 4 mins until the kale begins to crisp and wilt to half its size. Set aside.
- Adjust the heat so the water is at a rolling boil, then poach your eggs for 2 mins. Meanwhile, toast the bread.
- Remove the poached eggs with a slotted spoon and top each piece of toast with half the kale, an egg, the cherry tomatoes and feta

FRIED EGG FLORENTINE TOASTIES

Prep: 10 Mins - Cook: 10 Mins

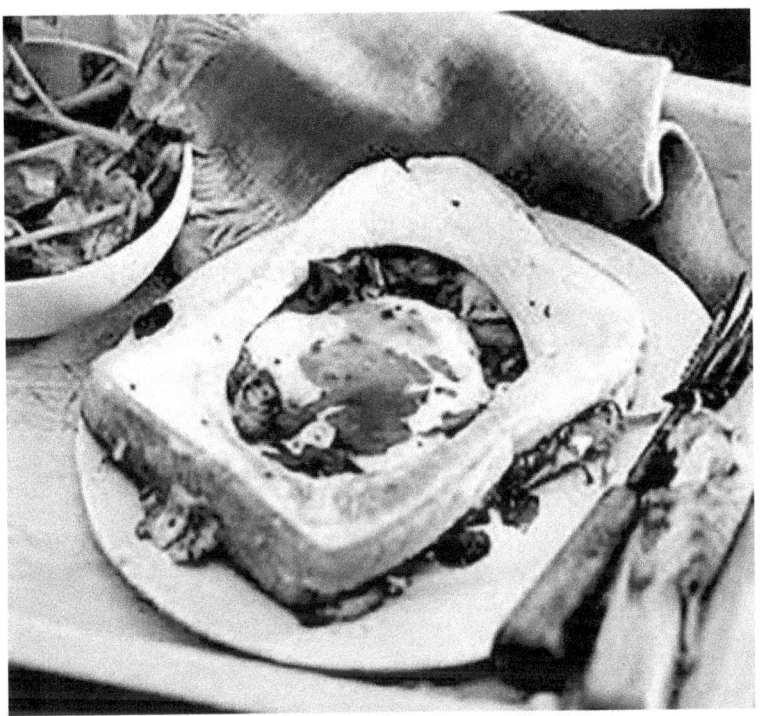

Ingredients

- » 2 slices of white bread knob of butter
- » 25g cheddar, grated
- » small handful baby spinach
- » 1 tbsp olive oil
- » 1 medium egg
- » sriracha hot sauce, to serve
- » extra spinach or watercress, to serve

Preparation

- Remove the centre of both slices of bread with the rim of a drinking glass or a cookie cutter. Spread each slice with a little butter and top both with the cheddar and torn spinach leaves – pack as much cheese and spinach on as you can. Heat a large non-stick pan over a medium heat and drizzle in the oil.
- Once the pan is hot, sandwich the bread together. Using a fish slice, place in the pan and press down to brown. Cook for 4-5 mins on a medium heat until the cheese begins to melt.
- Flip the sandwich over and crack the egg into the hole in the middle. Cover the pan with a lid to cook the egg through for 3-4 mins. Transfer to a plate, drizzle over some sriracha and serve with spinach or watercress on the side.

Apple Pie Overnight Oats

Prep Time: 10 mins - Total Time: 10 mins

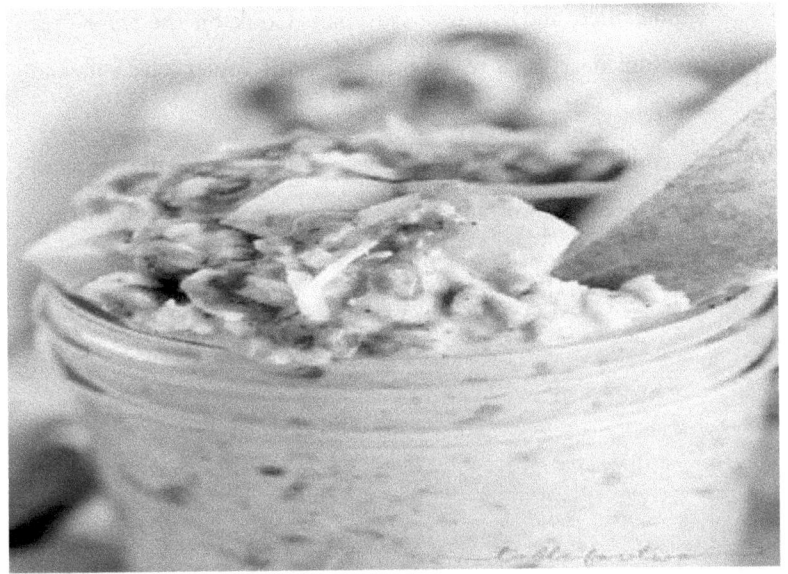

Ingredients

- 1 apple thinly sliced
- 2 Tbsp brown sugar 30 g
- 2 Tbsp almond butter 30 g
- ½ tsp ground cinnamon
- 1 tsp lemon juice 5 mL
- Pinch of salt
- 1 cup oats 150 g
- ½ cup milk 120 mL, can use dairy-free
- 2 Tbsp raisins 30 g

Preparation

- » Apples: Add sliced apple, sugar, almond butter, cinnamon, lemon juice, and salt to a saucepan. Cook on the stove over medium heat for 8 to 10 mins, or until apples have softened some.
- » Assemble: Spoon oats into two bowls or jars. Evenly top with apple mixture, milk, and raisins (you do not need to stir). Cover with a lid or plastic wrap and set in the refrigerator 6 hours (or overnight). Serve cold or heated in the microwave.

BANANA PEANUT BUTTER TORTILLA

10 Mins Prep Time - 10 Mins Total Time

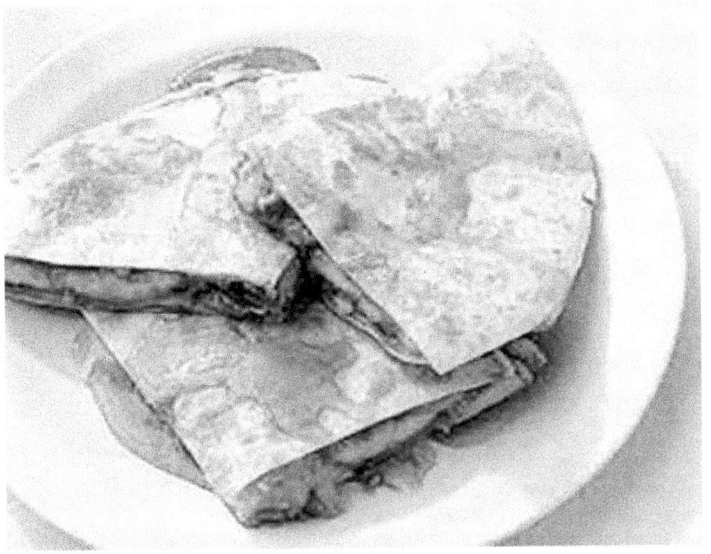

Ingredients

- 1 tortilla
- 12 tablespoons peanut butter
- 10 slices of banana
- 1 teaspoon organic honey
- Sprinkle of nutmeg powder

Preparation

- Heat a skillet and toast the tortilla for a mins on each side.
- Take it off the skillet and put it on a plate.
- Spread peanut butter on it evenly.
- Add the banana slices, honey, and nutmeg powder.
- Roll it or just fold it like a taco and enjoy!

Apple Carrot Muffin

Prep Time: 20 mins - Cook Time: 25 mins - Total Time: 45 mins

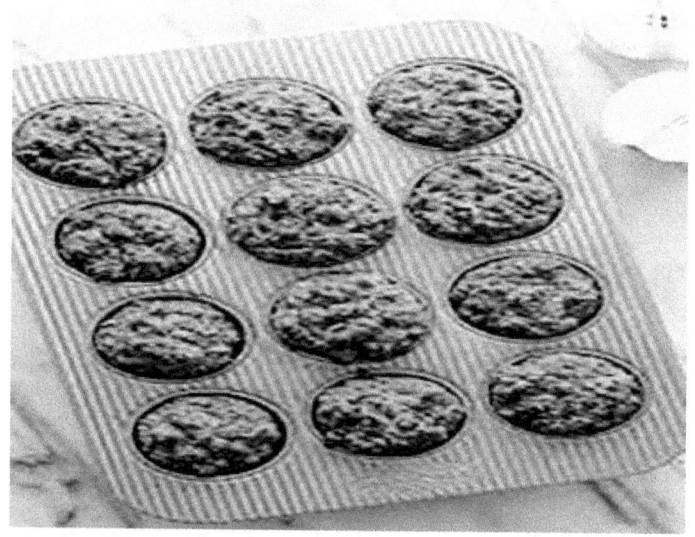

Ingredients

- » 1 ¼ cups flour
- » 1 ¾ cups oats bran
- » ¾ cup buttermilk
- » ¾ cup peeled and chopped apple
- » ¾ cup grated carrot
- » ⅔ cup brown sugar
- » ½ cup canola oil
- » 1 ½ teaspoons baking soda
- » ½ teaspoon salt
- » ¼ chopped walnuts
- » 1 teaspoon cinnamon powder

Preparation

- Mix oatmeal cereal, flour, sugar, baking soda, cinnamon, and salt in a bowl.
- Beat Canola oil and buttermilk in another bowl.
- Gently pour the wet ingredients into the bowl containing the dry ingredients.
- Now add the apples, carrots, and walnuts. Mix well.
- Preheat the oven to 200 degrees Celsius.
- Line muffin tray with paper liners.
- Put a spoonful of the batter into each muffin cup in the tray.
- Bake for 20-25 mins.
- Check by poking a toothpick in the center of the muffin. If it comes out clean, your muffins are ready.
- Cool them before eating.

Quinoa & Black Bean Breakfast for Weight Loss

Active: 20 mins - Total: 6 hrs. 35 mins

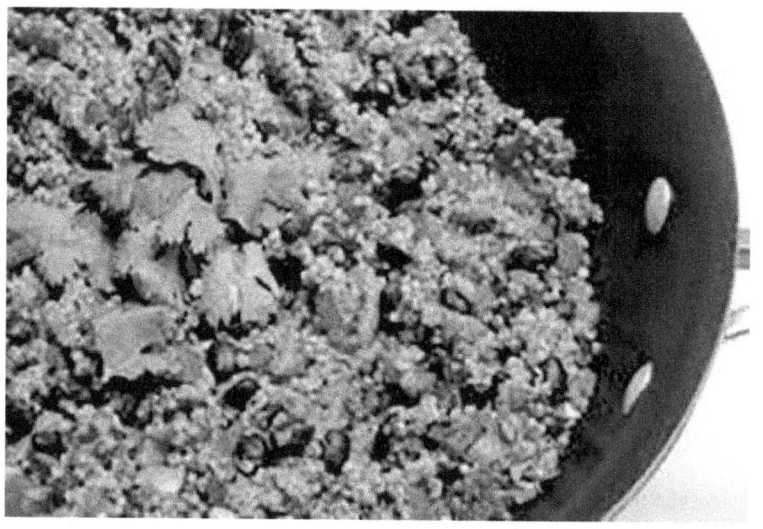

Ingredients

- ⅔ cup quinoa
- 1 tablespoon rice bran oil
- ¼ cup chopped onion
- 1 cup frozen corn kernels
- 1 can black beans
- 1 teaspoon chopped garlic
- ¼ teaspoon cayenne pepper
- 1 teaspoon cumin powder
- 1 ½ cup vegetable broth
- Handful of cilantro
- Salt to taste

Preparation

- Heat a pan and add rice bran oil.
- Add the onions and garlic and cook till the onions are translucent.
- Now stir in the quinoa, cayenne pepper, cumin powder, and vegetable broth.
- Cover and simmer till the mix comes to a boil.
- Add salt, black beans, and corn kernels and cook till the broth is absorbed.
- Transfer the cooked quinoa black bean to a plate and garnish with cilantro.

BUCKWHEAT WAFFLES
GLUTEN FREE BREAKFAST

Prep Time: 10 Mins - Cook Time: 10 Mins - Total Time: 20 Mins

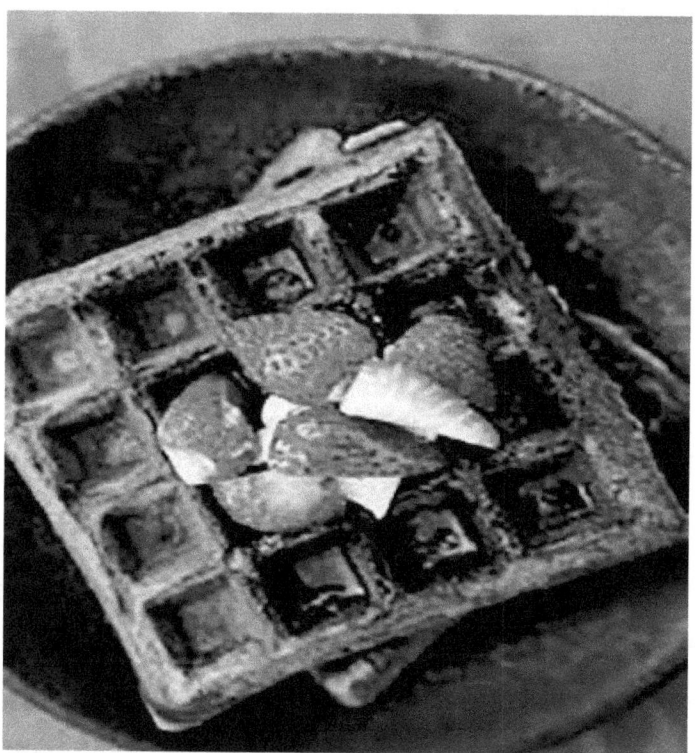

Ingredients

- » 1 cup buckwheat flour
- » 1 egg
- » ¼ cup coconut oil
- » 1 cup almond milk
- » 1 tablespoon coconut sugar
- » ¼ teaspoon cinnamon powder

- » 1 teaspoon baking powder
- » 1 teaspoon baking soda
- » 1 cup milk
- » 1 cup yogurt
- » ¼ cup water
- » ½ teaspoon salt
- » 4 banana slices
- » 2 tablespoons maple syrup
- » 2 tablespoons peanut butter

Preparation

- » Turn your waffle maker and set it on medium.
- » Mix buckwheat flour, baking soda, baking powder, salt, and cinnamon.
- » Separate the egg white and beat it using an electric egg beater or whisker.
- » Add the sugar while you beat the egg. Beat it till you get soft peaks.
- » In a bowl, whisk egg yolk, water, milk, and yogurt.
- » Pour the wet mix into the dry mix and fold the beaten egg whites into the batter.
- » Pour this batter into your waffle maker and cook until the waffle maker indicator shows that the waffle is cooked.
- » Gently push the waffle out using a fork.
- » Serve with maple syrup and peanut butter.

Zucchini Muffins

Prep Time: 15 Mins - Cook Time: 25 Mins

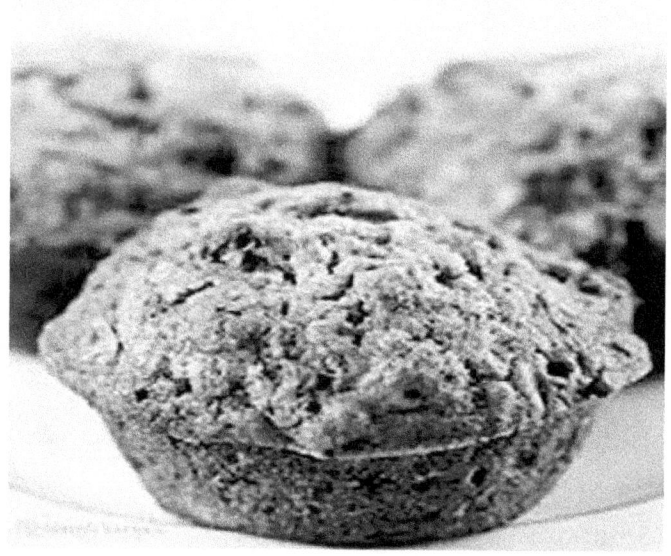

Ingredients

- 1 cup peeled and grated zucchini
- ¾ cup all-purpose flour
- 1 egg
- ¼ cup chopped raisins
- ¼ cup rice bran oil
- ½ cup brown sugar
- ¼ teaspoon baking soda
- ¼ teaspoon baking powder
- ¼ teaspoon salt
- ½ cup chopped walnut
- ¼ teaspoon ground cinnamon

Preparation

- Mix the flour, sugar, salt, baking soda, baking powder, and cinnamon powder in a bowl.
- Add the oil and egg to the mix and combine.
- Fold in the raisins and zucchini.
- Preheat the oven.
- Grease a muffin tray and add 1-2 tablespoons of the batter in each greased cup.
- Bake for 25 mins at 350 degrees Celsius.
- Cool for 5 mins before eating.

Chapter 7
LUNCH RECIPES

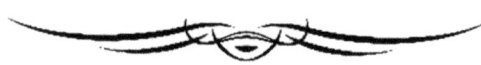

EASY HUEVOS RANCHEROS
Rep: 3 Mins - Cook: 7 Mins

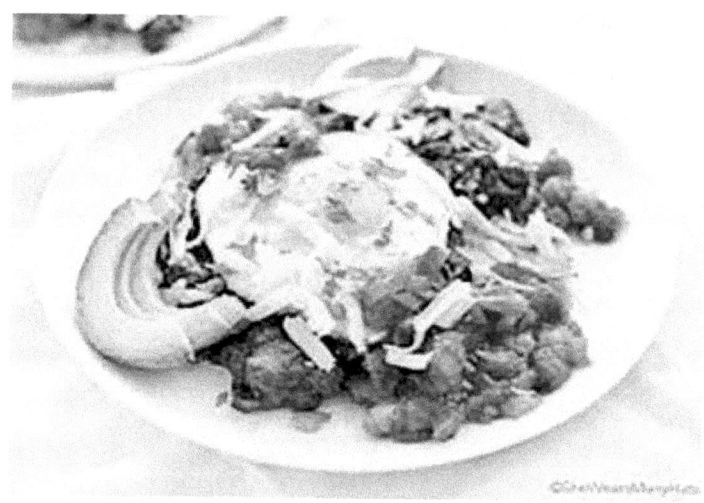

Ingredients

- » 1 tbsp vegetable oil or sunflower oil
- » 1 corn tortilla wrap
- » 1 egg
- » 200g can black beans, drained
- » juice ½ lime
- » ½ ripe avocado, peeled and sliced
- » 50g feta, crumbled
- » hot chili sauce (we like sriracha)

Preparation

- » Heat the oil in a frying pan over a high heat. Add the tortilla and fry for 1-2 mins on each side until crisping at the edges. Transfer to a plate.
- » Crack the egg into the pan and cook to your liking. Meanwhile, tip the beans into a bowl, season and add a squeeze of lime, then lightly mash with a fork.
- » Spread the beans over the tortilla, top with the egg, avocado, feta and chilli sauce. Squeeze over a little more lime juice just before eating.

Seasoned Brown Lentils

Prep Time: 5 Mins - Cook Time: 20 Mins

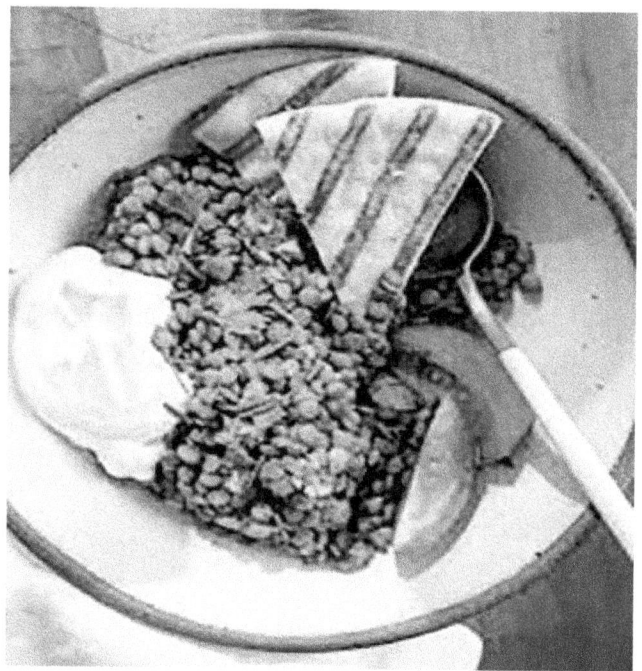

Ingredients

- For the brown lentils
- 4 cups vegetable broth (or water, or a combination of both)
- 1 1/2 cups brown lentils
- 1 1/2 teaspoons onion powder
- 1 1/2 teaspoons paprika
- 1 teaspoon oregano
- 1/2 teaspoon garlic powder
- 1/2 teaspoon black pepper
- 3/4 teaspoon kosher salt

Preparation

- » Place all Ingredients in a large saucepan. (If you're planning to cook them without seasoning to use in a separate recipe, omit the spices, salt, and pepper.)
- » Bring to a rapid simmer, then reduce the heat and simmer for about 20 to 25 mins until the lentils are tender but still hold their shape. There will be some leftover broth but the lentils will soak it up as they sit and become perfectly moist. Taste and add another pinch of salt if you'd like. Serve warm. (Storage info: Leftovers can be stored in the refrigerator; reheat on the stovetop.)

The Runner's Sandwich

Prep Time 5 mins - Cook Time 5 mins - Total Time 10 mins

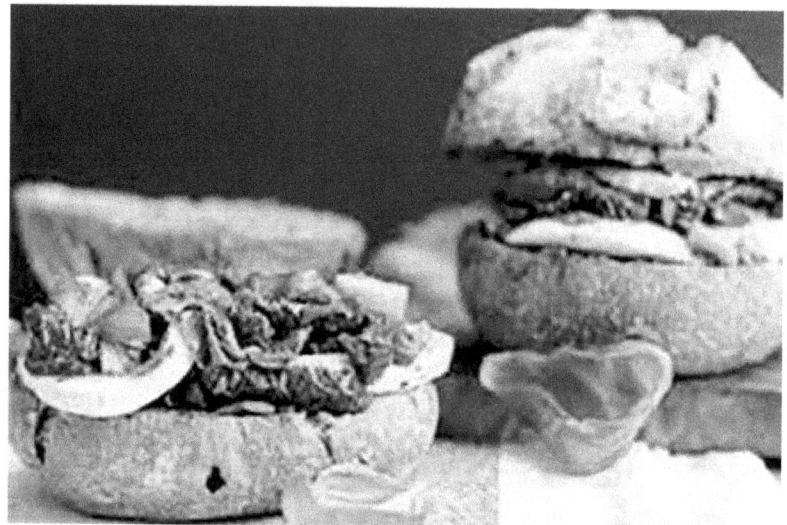

Ingredients

- 4 slices bread (whole wheat)
- ½ ball mozzarella (cottage cheese also goes great!)
- ¼ cup sun-dried tomatoes in oil
- 2 tbsp olives
- 2 tsp capers (can be made without if unavailable)
- ¼ cup basil, fresh (dried basil is also fine, ¼ cup = 1 tsp)
- salt and pepper to taste
- Optional:
- 2 tbsp olive oil
- 1 tsp chili flakes
- 1 small handful oregano, fresh (1 small handful fresh = ½ tsp dried)

Preparation

- Roughly chop the cheese, tomatoes, olives and capers and throw into a mixing bowl.
- Add the herbs, salt and pepper.
- Use a fork to mix up and mash the ingredients a little - not too much, we just want to get those flavours circulating.
- If you're using very soft bread then pop it in the toaster/pan without oil for a mins or so - not to toast it, just to harden the outside. If the bread is already a hard type, we're good to go.
- Spread the mix on the bottom slices, add the other slices on top. Squish down.
- Now comes the oil part - if you're exercising a lot you're gonna need all that extra fatty olive oil. If you're not, that's your call. Either way, it tastes great.
- Heat the pan (with or without the oil) and put the sandwich in. Put a lid on the pan if you have one, don't stress too much if you don't. Cook for 3 or 4 mins, squishing down with a spatula occasionally, then flip and cook the other side the same way. Both outsides should be nice and crispy, the insides melting together.

Hummus and Veggie Roll Ups

Prep: 10 Mins

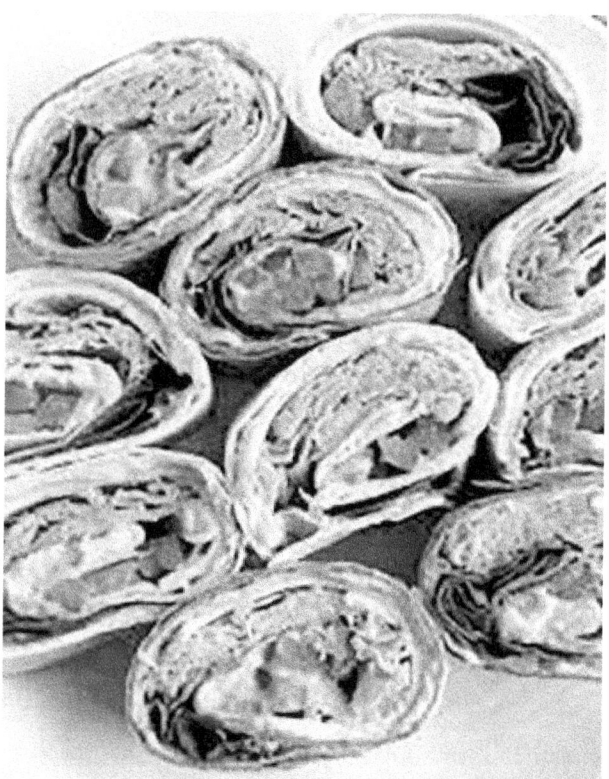

Ingredients

- 4 large Dole® carrots
- 1 large head Dole® broccoli
- 1 small head Dole® cauliflower
- 3 green onions
- 8 8-inch whole wheat or multigrain tortillas
- 8 ounces (1 cup) high quality hummus*, purchased or homemade

Preparation

- Peel and shred the carrots, using a julienne peeler or box grater. Slice the tops off of the broccoli and the cauliflower into very small pieces (as shown in the photograph). Thinly slice the green onions.
- Spread about 2 tablespoons of hummus onto a tortilla in a thin layer. Sprinkle another thin layer vegetables on top, taking care not to overfill and leaving the very top of the tortilla without vegetables (as shown in the photograph). Starting from the bottom of the circle, tightly roll the tortilla; as you roll to the top, the vegetables will naturally move up and distribute evenly through the rollup. Use a serrated knife to cut the roll into 6 or 8 pieces. If desired, spear with toothpicks. Refrigerate until serving.

Coleslaw & Swiss Melt Sandwich

Prep Time: 15 mins - Cook Time: 5 mins

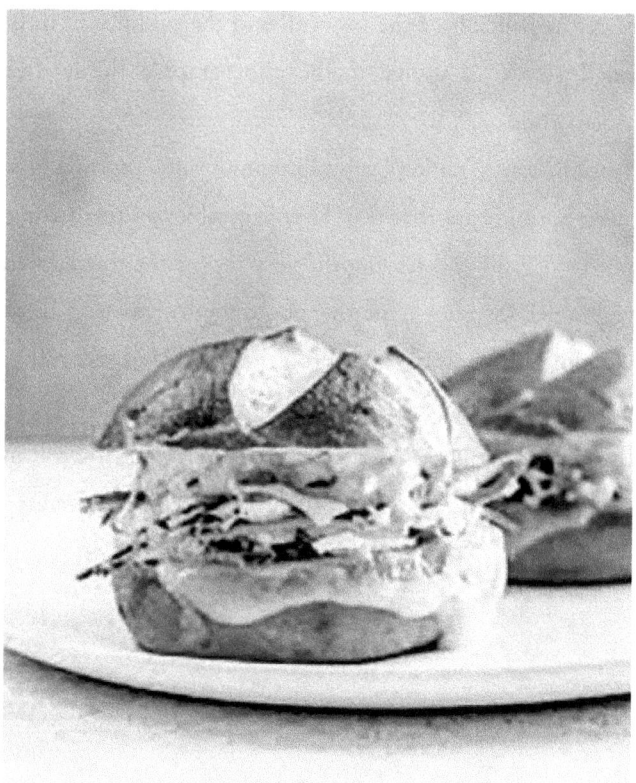

Ingredients

- » 2 cups Best Coleslaw Recipe or Red Cabbage Slaw
- » 1/4 cup Easy Russian Dressing
- » 4 slices Swiss cheese
- » 4 pretzel rolls or 8 slices artisan or rye bread

Preparation

» Place the bottoms of the pretzel buns on a baking sheet and place a slice of Swiss cheese on top. Place the tops of the buns on the sheet as well. Broil for about 4 to 5 mins until the cheese is melted and the buns are toasted. OR

Chickpea Salad

Prep Time 10 Mins - Total Time 10 Mins

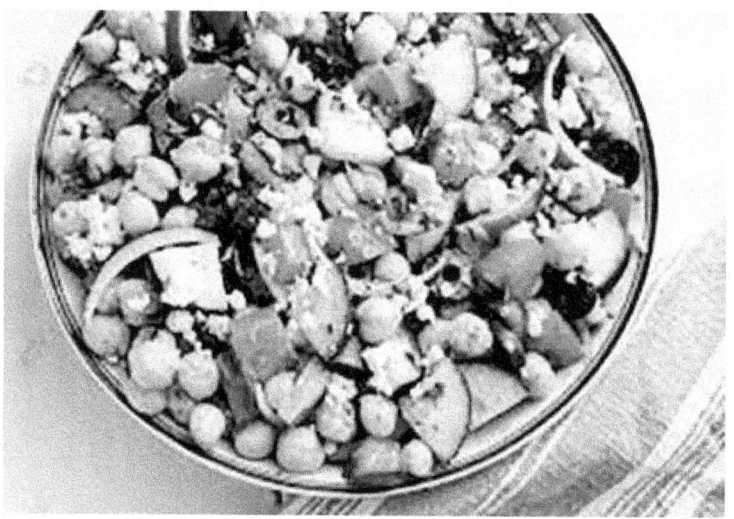

Ingredients

- » 15-ounce can chickpeas
- » 1/4 cup bell pepper, diced
- » 1/4 cup English cucumber, chopped
- » 1/2 tablespoon olive oil
- » 1/2 tablespoon red wine vinegar
- » 1/2 teaspoon kosher salt
- » 1/2 teaspoon smoked paprika
- » Fresh ground pepper
- » 1 pinch celery seed or fresh torn herbs (parsley, dill, basil, etc), optional

Preparation

- » Drain and rinse the chickpeas.
- » Dice the bell pepper. Chop the cucumber (peel it if you're using a standard cucumber; English cucumber doesn't need to be peeled).
- » In a bowl, mix together all Ingredients. Taste and add salt as desired.

DOMINATE

Glowing Green Hummus

Prep Time: 15 mins - Cook Time: 0 mins

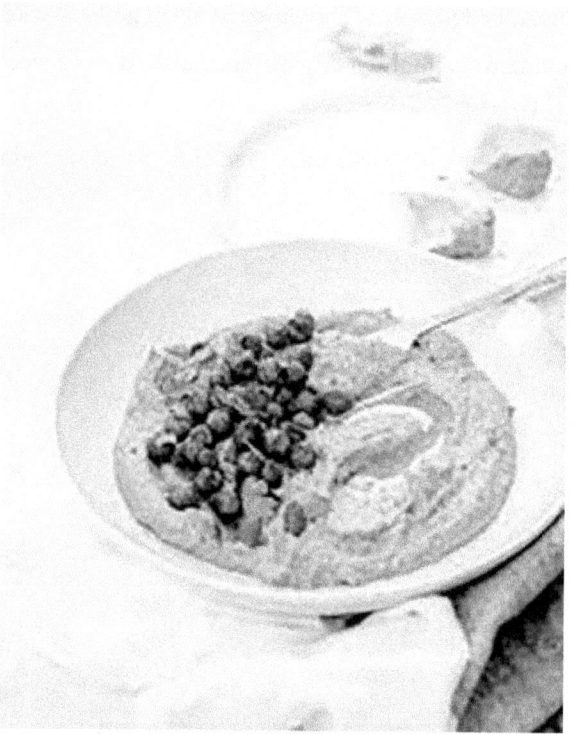

Ingredients

- For the green hummus
- 1 small garlic clove
- 1 15-ounce can chickpeas
- 1/4 cup lime juice (2 limes)
- 2 green onions
- 1/2 cup packed cilantro leaves and tender stems
- 2 cups baby spinach leaves

- 1/4 cup tahini
- 1/4 teaspoon cumin
- 3/4 teaspoon kosher salt
- 1/4 cup aquafaba (can liquid from the chickpeas), plus more as needed
- For the garnish
- Olive oil, cilantro leaves, Crispy Chickpeas

Preparation

- Peel the garlic. Drain the chickpeas into a liquid measuring cup. Juice the limes. Chop the green onions into 1 inch pieces, including the greens.
- Add the garlic, cilantro, green onion, and spinach, to the bowl of a food processor and process until finely chopped. Add chickpeas, lime juice, tahini, cumin, kosher salt, and water from the chickpea can (aquafaba). Puree for 30 seconds, then scrape down the bowl. Taste. If necessary, add 1 to 2 tablespoons aquafaba. Puree for 1 to 2 mins to come to a creamy consistency. Store refrigerated for 7 to 10 days.
- If desired, top the hummus with cilantro leaves, a drizzle of olive oil, and Crispy Chickpeas. Serve with veggies, pita bread, or crackers (like these homemade crackers!)

Ricotta & White Bean Fancy Toast

Prep Time: 15 mins - Cook Time: 15 mins

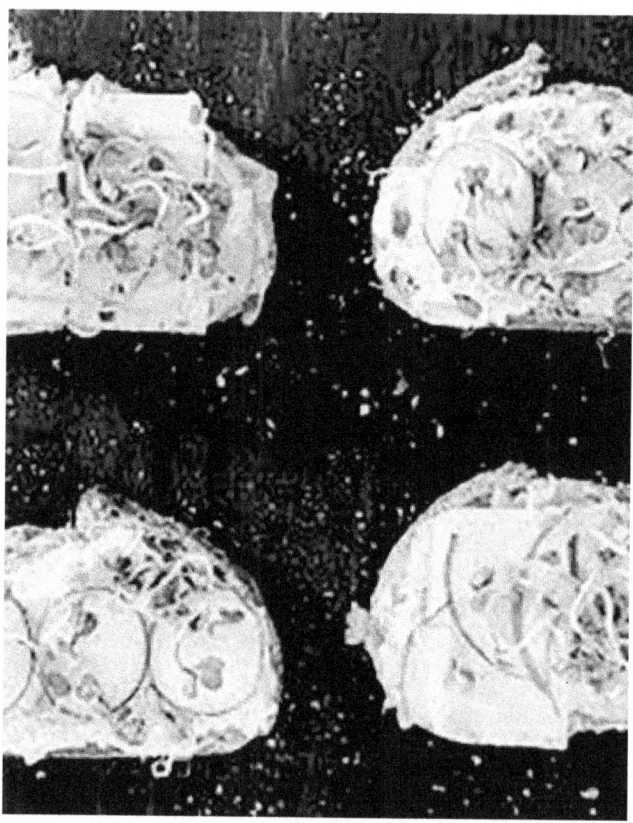

Ingredients

- For the ricotta & radish fancy toast
- 1 cup fresh ricotta cheese
- 1/2 teaspoon kosher salt, divided
- 4 to 5 radishes
- 1/2 cup sprouts (radish, alfalfa, etc.)
- 4 slices good quality bread

- » Fresh ground pepper
- » For the white bean Havarti fancy toast
- » 15-ounce can cannellini beans
- » 1/2 teaspoon kosher salt
- » 1 tablespoon olive oil
- » ½ red onion
- » 1/2 cup sprouts (radish, alfalfa, etc)
- » 8 slices dill Havarti cheese
- » 4 slices good quality bread
- » Fresh ground pepper

Preparation

- » Make the ricotta spread: In a small bowl, stir together the ricotta cheese, kosher salt, and fresh ground pepper.
- » Thinly slice the radishes. Spread 4 bread slices with seasoned ricotta spread, then top with radishes, a sprinkle of kosher salt, and sprouts.
- » Make the white bean spread: Drain and rinse the white beans. In a small bowl, stir together beans with the kosher salt, olive oil, and fresh ground pepper. Mash together with a fork until a thick spread form.
- » Thinly slice the red onion. Rinse the onion slices under cold water several times to mellow the flavor. Spread another 4 bread slices with white bean spread, then top with Havarti cheese, red onion slices, and sprouts.

Perfect Hard-Boiled Eggs (How Long to Boil)

Prep Time 1 Mins - Cook Time 7 Mins - Total Time 8 Mins

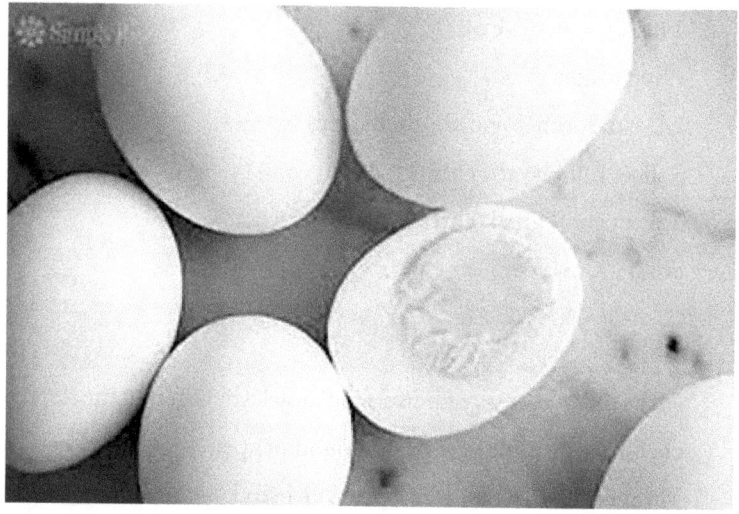

Ingredients

- » 12 large eggs (older eggs peel better than fresh)
- » Ice

Preparation

- » Place 12 eggs in the bottom of a large pot and and cover with water 1 inch above the eggs.
- » Bring the water to a boil, gently stirring the eggs several times.
- » As soon as the water boils, remove the pot from the heat, cover, and let the eggs sit for 15 mins (13 mins for small eggs or 17 mins extra large eggs). Prepare a bowl of ice water.

» After 15 mins, place the eggs in the ice water and allow them to cool completely (about 15 mins). Peel immediately, or store in the fridge for 4 to 5 days.

Avocado Toast with Egg

PREP TIME: 5 mins - COOK TIME: 5 mins - TOTAL TIME: 10 mins

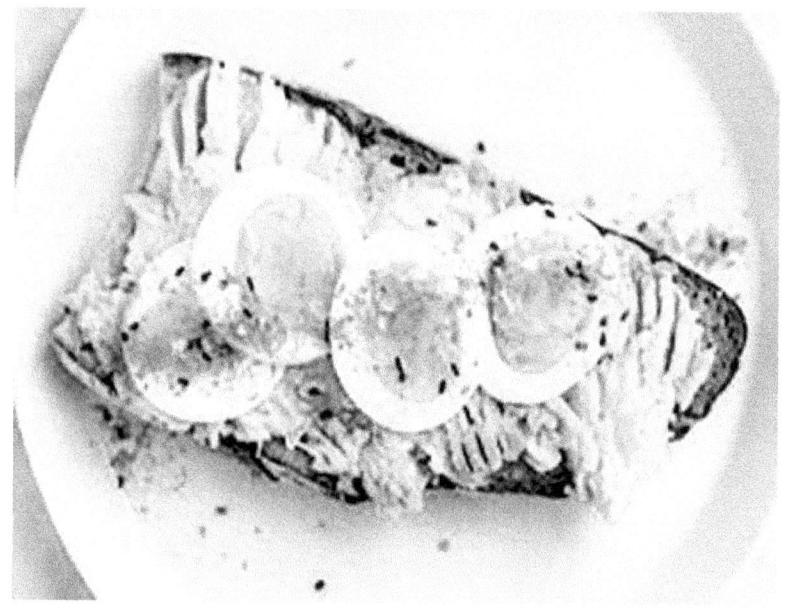

Ingredients

- For the turmeric poached egg*
- ¼ cup distilled white vinegar
- 2 teaspoons ground turmeric
- 2 large eggs
- For the avocado toast
- 2 thick slices artisan bread or Homemade Bread
- 1 avocado
- 1 to 2 radishes
- Black sesame seeds
- Chunky sea salt

Preparation

- In a large saucepan, pour a few inches of water and bring it to a boil. Reduce to a gentle simmer and stir in the vinegar and turmeric.
- Crack an egg into a small bowl, then gently slide the egg into water. Wait about 30 seconds, then add the next egg. Allow to simmer for about 3 mins, until the whites are set but the yolks are runny.
- Line a plate with a paper towel. Remove the eggs from the pan using a slotted spoon, then allow them to drain while preparing the toast. (Throughout the process, take care with the turmeric water, as it can stain clothing.)
- Remove the avocado pit, scoop it out of the peel, and mash it with some salt using a fork. Spread it on the bread slices, then top with radishes, sesame seeds, and sea salt.

Sweet Potato Noodles Stir-Fry

Prep Time 5 mins - Cook Time 15 mins - Total Time 20 mins

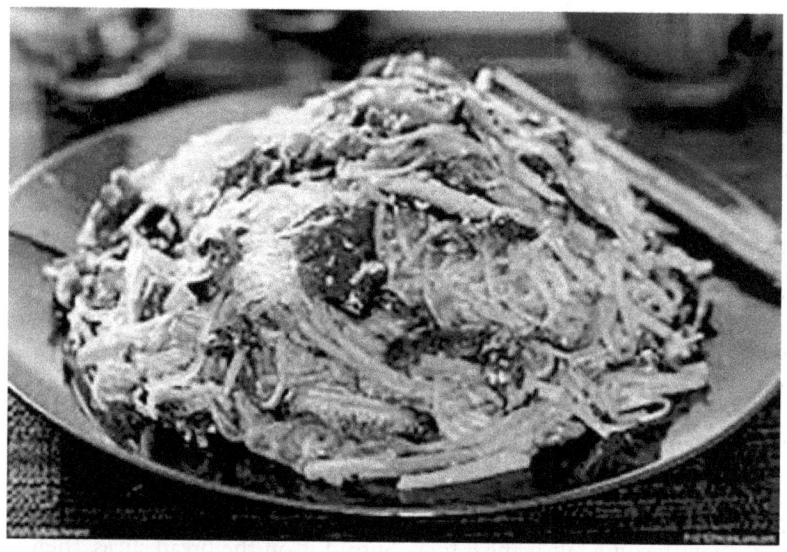

Ingredients

- 1 medium onion finely diced
- 1 sweet pepper diced
- 4 cloves garlic minced
- 2 cups broccoli florets
- 2 tablespoons olive oil
- 2 medium sweet potatoes spiralized
- 2 tablespoons soy sauce
- Salt and pepper to taste

Preparation

- In a large skillet over medium-high heat, saute onion, pepper, garlic, and broccoli in olive oil until vegetables are just tender, about 7-10 mins.
- Stir in sweet potato noodles and soy sauce and stir occasionally until noodles are softened, an additional 7-10 mins. Season noodles with salt and pepper to taste and serve hot. Enjoy!

Ricotta and Spinach Calzones

Prep Time: 15 mins - Cook Time: 15 mins - Total Time: 30 mins

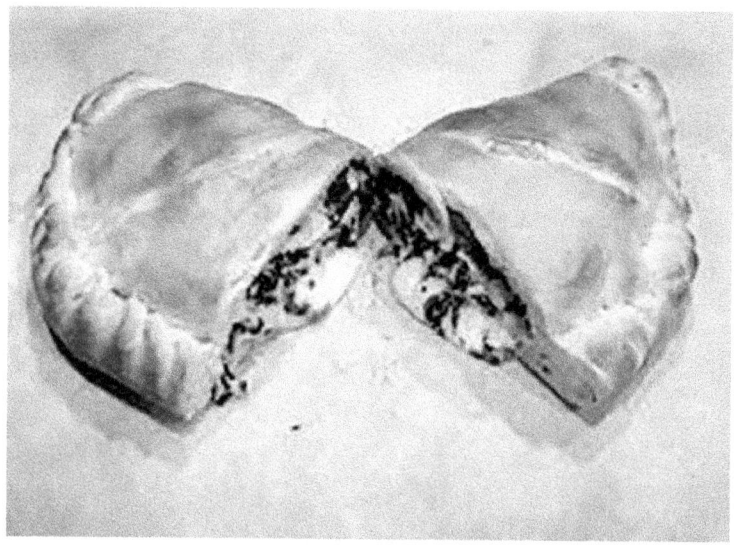

Ingredients

- 10 ounces frozen chopped spinach, thawed and squeezed dry
- 8 ounces ricotta cheese
- 4 ounces mozzarella cheese, shredded
- 1 ounce Parmesan cheese, grated
- 1 tablespoon olive oil (affiliate)
- 1 large egg, lightly beaten with 2 tablespoons water, plus 1 large egg yolk
- 1 teaspoon garlic powder
- 1 1/2 teaspoons minced fresh oregano
- 1/8 teaspoon red pepper flakes
- 1 teaspoon salt
- 1 lb pizza dough

Preparation

- Preheat oven to 500 degrees.
- Combine spinach, ricotta, mozzarella, oil, egg yolk, garlic powder, oregano, pepper flakes, and salt in a large bowl.
- Place dough on lightly floured surface and divide into 4 even pieces.
- With a rolling pin or your hands, flatten each piece into a 7 inch round on a piece of parchment paper.
- Spread 1/4 of spinach filling evenly over half of each dough round, making sure to leave a 1 inch border around the edge.
- Brush the edges with the egg wash and then fold the other half of the dough circle over spinach mixture, leaving the bottom 1/2 inch border uncovered.
- Press edges of dough together and pinch with fingers to seal.
- With a sharp knife, cut 5 steam vents in top of calzones and brush tops with remaining egg wash.
- Transfer calzones onto parchment lined baking sheet and bake for 8 mins, brush with any remaining egg wash and sprinkle with grated parmesan, then bake for another 7 mins.
- Move to wire rack and let cool for 5 mins before serving.

Lentil Tortilla Soup

Prep Time 10 Mins - Cook Time 15 Mins - Total Time 50 Mins

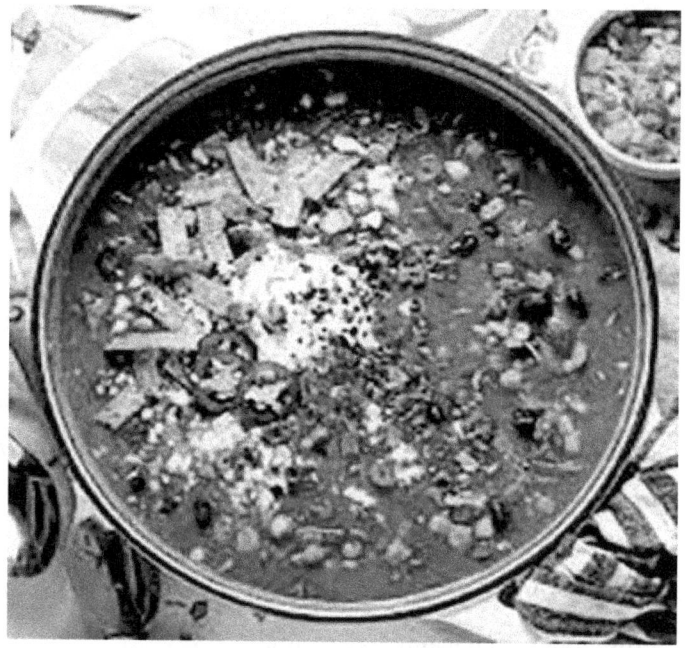

Ingredients

- 1 cup diced onion
- 1 tsp avocado oil (or olive oil)
- 1 bell pepper diced
- 1 jalapeno pepper diced
- 2.5 cups vegetable broth (or chicken broth if needed)
- 15 oz canned tomato sauce or crushed tomatoes
- 1/2 cup mild or medium salsa verde (or your favorite salsa!)
- 1 TBSP tomato paste
- 15 oz can black beans (drained + rinsed)

- » 15 oz can pinto beans (drained + rinsed)
- » 1 cup corn (fresh, canned, or frozen)
- » 3/4 cup dried red lentils
- » 1/2 tsp chili powder
- » 1/2 tsp garlic powder
- » 1/2 tsp cumin
- » 1/4 tsp cayenne pepper
- » 1/4-1/2 cup heavy cream

Preparation

- » First, chop your veggies and measure out the Ingredients.
- » Next add everything but the heavy cream your toppings.
- » This includes bell pepper, jalapeño, corn, lentils, black beans, pinto beans, broth, tomato sauce, tomato paste, salsa verde, and all your herbs + spices. Toss them in and set IP to high pressure for 15 mins.
- » Allow natural pressure release.
- » Stir in the cream, add all your favorite toppings, and enjoy!

Cold Spicy Peanut Sesame Noodles

Prep time:1 hr. - cook time:25 mins - total time:1 hr. 25 mins

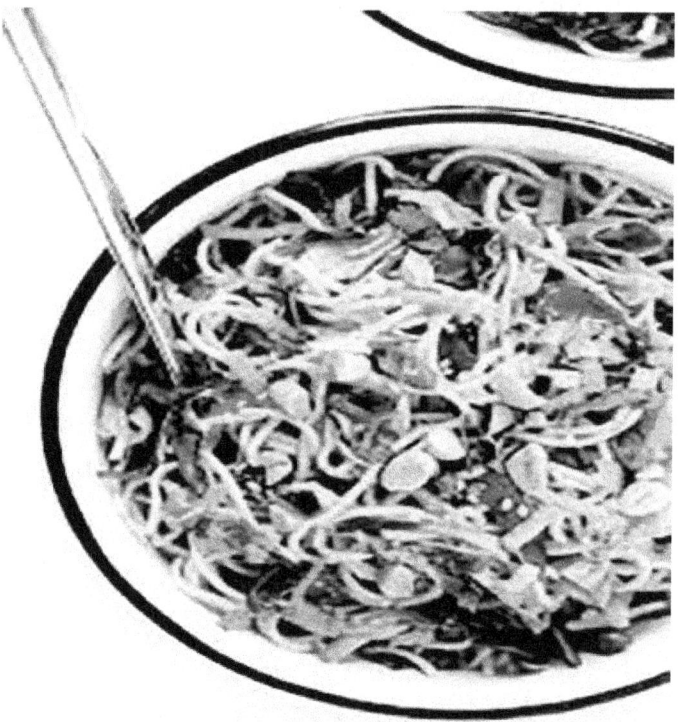

Ingredients

- 3/4 cup to 1-pound dried spaghetti noodles, or Asian rice noodles
- 2/3 cup water
- 1/3 cup smooth peanut butter
- 1/4 cup low sodium soy sauce
- 1/4 cup seasoned rice vinegar
- 3 tbsp dark brown sugar, packed

- 1/4 cup roasted peanut oil
- 2 tbsp toasted sesame seeds, plus more for topping
- 3 tsp chili garlic sauce
- 1 tsp sesame oil
- 1: 1- inch piece of ginger, peeled
- 1 clove small of garlic
- Fresh scallions, chopped, for topping

Preparation

- In a large stockpot, bring water to boil then add spaghetti noodles and cook according to box. Drain well when done.
- In a jar of a blender, combine water, peanut butter, soy sauce, rice vinegar, brown sugar, peanut oil, sesame seeds, chili garlic sauce, sesame oil, ginger, and garlic. Process until smooth.
- After pasta is done cooking and drained, add to a large glass bowl. Pour the peanut sesame sauce over the noodles and toss to coat. The mixture/sauce will be very runny and it will look like you made way too much. Trust me, once you pop it in the fridge, the sauce sets up and it's perfect :)
- Cover and refrigerate for at least one hour - the longer, the better. I had mine in there for at least three. I love when it's super cold and the sauce is nice and thick.
- Toss noodles again prior to serving. Top with fresh scallions and sesame seeds.

Spinach, Artichoke and Goat Cheese Quiche

Prep Time: 20 Mins - Cook Time: 40 Mins

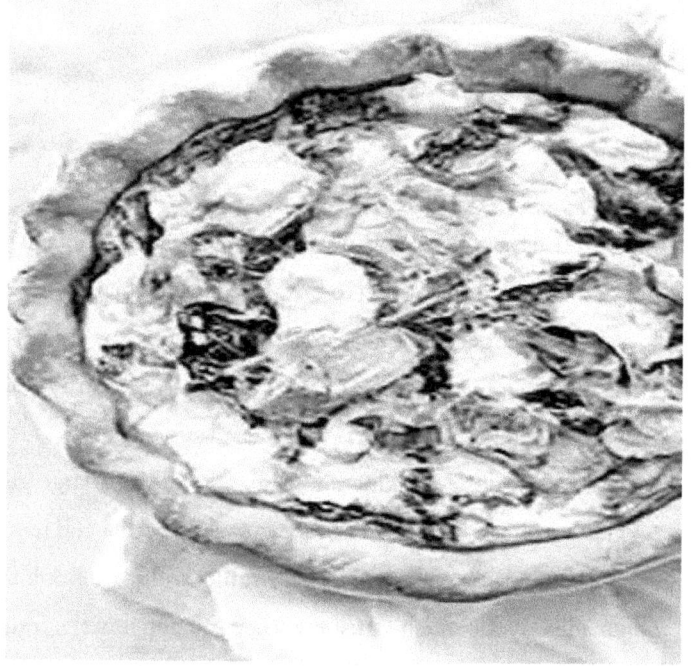

Ingredients

- 1 store-bought refrigerator pie dough or this homemade pie dough
- 1 tablespoon butter
- 1 leek thinly sliced, white and light green parts only
- 1 cup frozen artichoke hearts thawed and quartered
- 1 1/2 cups fresh spinach
- 1/2 teaspoon kosher salt

- » 6 eggs
- » 1 1/4 cups Almond Breeze Almond Milk Original Unsweetened
- » 1/2 teaspoon ground mustard
- » 1/4 teaspoon nutmeg
- » 2 ounces goat cheese

Preparation

- » Preheat the oven to 375 degrees F.
- » Roll out the pie dough and line a 9-inch pie pan with the dough then place in the refrigerator to keep chilled.
- » Melt the butter in a skillet over medium heat. Add the leeks and cook until the leeks soften, about 5 mins, stirring often. Add the artichoke hearts to the pan and cook for another 2 mins or so. Stir in the spinach, season with kosher salt and remove from the heat and stir so the warm vegetables wilt the spinach and set aside to cool.
- » Whisk the eggs and Almond milk with the mustard and nutmeg. Pull the pie tin from the refrigerator and fill the bottom with the cooked vegetables. Top with half of the goat cheese. Pour the egg mixture over the vegetables and top with more goat cheese.
- » Bake for 45-55 mins or until the egg is puffed and no longer jiggly. Remove from the oven and let rest for 10 mins. Serve warm or at room temperature.

Roasted Chickpea Gyros

Prep: 10 mins - Cook: 20 mins - Total: 30 mins

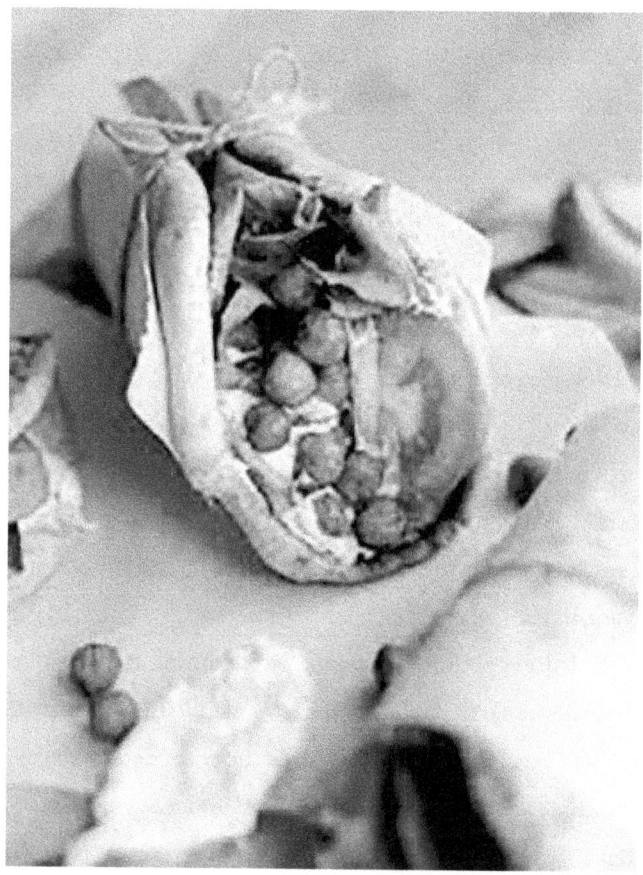

Ingredients

» 1 15 oz can chickpeas 425 g, 1 ½ cup-soaked chickpeas if starting from dry, drained and rinsed

» 1 Tbsp olive oil 15 mL

» 1 Tbsp paprika* 7 g

- 1 tsp ground black pepper 3 g
- 1/2 tsp cayenne pepper 1.5 g
- 1/4 tsp salt 1.5 g
- 4 pita flatbreads
- 1 cup tzatziki (click for recipe) 250 g, use ⅓ recipe if you're just making it for these gyros
- 1/4 red onion cut into strips
- 2 lettuce leaves roughly chopped
- 1 tomato sliced

Preparation

- Prep: Preheat oven to 400 degrees F (204 C). Pat dry chickpeas with paper towel, removing any skins that may come off. Gently toss chickpeas with oil, paprika, black pepper, cayenne pepper, and salt.
- Roast: Spread chickpeas onto a greased rimmed baking sheet and roast for about 20 mins, until lightly browned but not hard.
- Assemble: Spread some tzatziki onto one side of the pita, then sprinkle in ¼ of the chickpeas and add veggies. Fold in half and enjoy!

Crispy Baked Black Bean & Sweet Potato Tacos

Prep Time: 20 mins - Cook Time: 10 mins

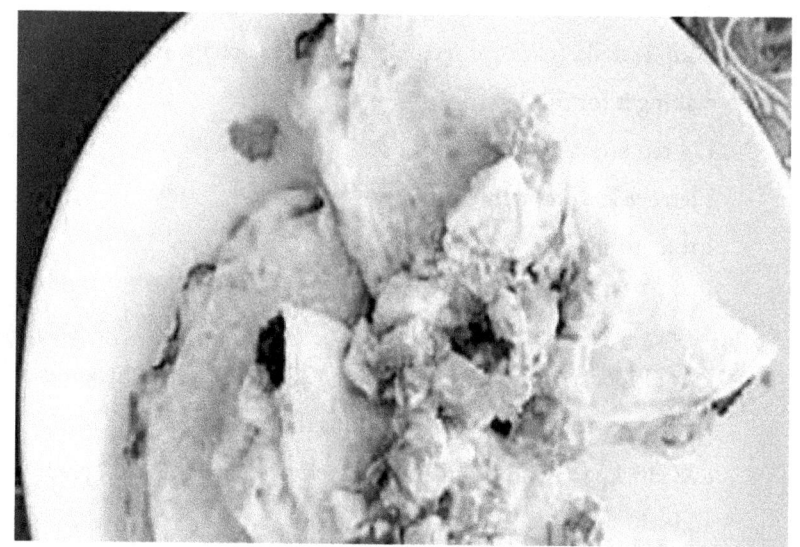

Ingredients

- » 1 cup refried black beans
- » 1 cup sweet potato puree, homemade or canned*
- » 1 cup grated cheese
- » 8 corn tortillas
- » Olive oil
- » 1 large avocado, diced
- » 1 tomato, small diced
- » 1/4 cup chopped red onion
- » 1 clove garlic, minced
- » 1 tablespoon chopped cilantro
- » Juice of 1 lime
- » Salt, to taste

Preparation

- Pre-heat oven to 450 F. Line a large baking sheet with parchment paper and brush with a small amount of olive oil. If corn tortillas aren't very pliable you may need to warm on the stove or microwave for about 5 seconds each before assembling tacos.
- Spread about 1 tablespoon of refried beans on half of the tortilla and top with 1 tablespoon sweet potato and a sprinkling of cheese. Fold tortilla over and repeat with remaining ingredients. Brush the top of each taco with a small amount of olive oil and bake for about 10 mins, flipping once.
- Make the avocado salsa while tacos are baking. Add all ingredients to a medium sized bowl and mix until combined.
- Let tacos cool for a few mins before eating and top with avocado salsa, if desired. Recipe serves 2-3 people but can easily be adapted to make more.

Vegetarian Lettuce Wraps

Total Time - 15 Mins

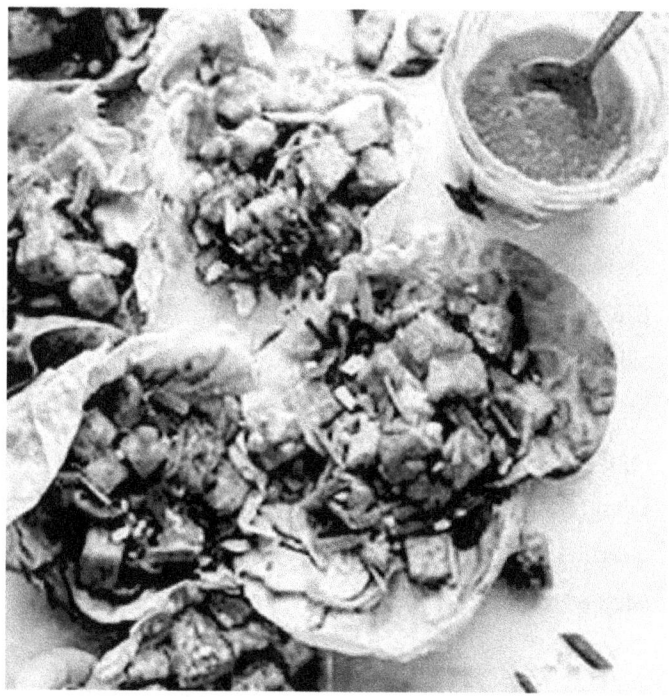

Ingredients

- 3 tablespoons hoisin sauce
- 3 tablespoons reduced-sodium soy sauce
- 2 tablespoons rice vinegar
- 1 teaspoon sesame oil
- 2 teaspoons canola oil - or grapeseed oil
- 1 package extra-firm tofu - (12- to 14-ounces), do not use silken
- 8 ounces baby belle cremini mushrooms - finely chopped
- 1 can water chestnuts - (8 ounces), drained and finely chopped

- » 2 cloves garlic - minced
- » 2 teaspoons freshly grated ginger
- » 1/4 teaspoon red pepper flakes - omit if sensitive to spice
- » 4 green onions - thinly sliced, divided
- » 8 large inner leaves romaine lettuce - from a romaine heart or butter lettuce leaves

Preparation

- » In a small bowl, stir together the hoisin, soy sauce, rice vinegar, and sesame oil. Set aside.
- » Press the tofu between paper towels to squeeze out as much liquid as possible. Refresh the paper towels and press again. Heat the 2 teaspoons canola oil in a large nonstick skillet over medium-high. Once the oil is hot, crumble in the tofu, breaking it into very small pieces as it cooks. Continue cooking for 5 mins, then add the diced mushrooms. Continue cooking until any remaining tofu liquid cooks off and the tofu starts to turn golden, about 3 mins more. Stir in the water chestnuts, garlic, ginger, red pepper flakes, and half of the green onions and cook until fragrant, about 30 seconds more.
- » Pour the sauce over the top of the tofu mixture and stir to coat. Cook just until you hear bubbling and the sauce is warmed through, 30 to 60 seconds.
- » Spoon the tofu mixture into individual lettuce leaves. Top with remaining green onions, grated carrots, and additional red pepper flakes as desired. Serve immediately.

Peanut Tofu Buddha Bowl

Prep Time: 20 Mins - Cook Time: 15 Mins - Total Time: 35 Mins

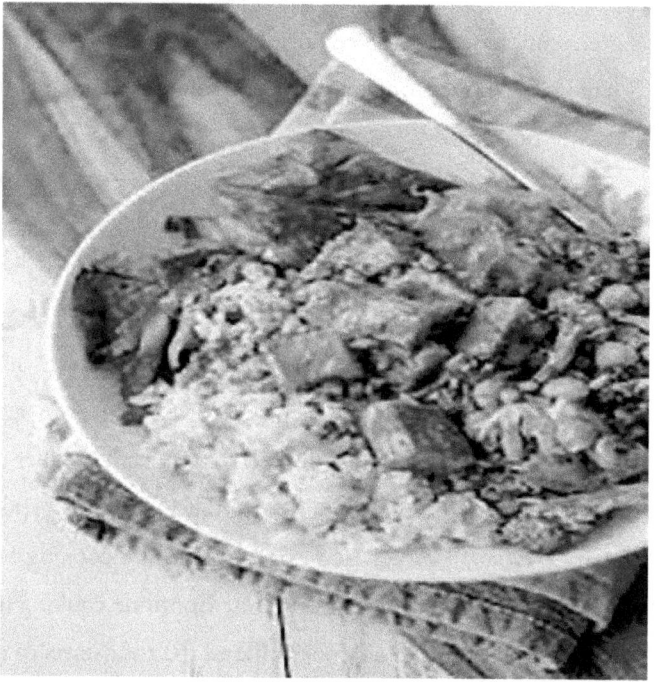

Ingredients

- Tofu Buddha Bowl
- 2 cups cooked brown rice
- 1 cups shredded carrots
- 2 cups spinach leaves
- 2 cups broccoli florets
- 2 teaspoons olive oil or additional sesame oil, divided
- 1 cup chickpeas (drained and rinsed, if using canned)
- salt/pepper

- 16 oz extra firm tofu, pressed and drained
- Peanut sauce
- 1–2 tablespoons toasted sesame oil
- 1/4 cup low sodium soy sauce
- 1/4 cup 100% pure maple syrup
- 2 teaspoons chili garlic sauce
- 1/4 cup creamy or crunchy peanut butter

Preparation

- Preheat the oven to 400 degrees F. Cube tofu and place in a single layer on a non-stick baking sheet and cook for 25 mins. If you aren't using a non-stick baking sheet, lightly spray with cooking spray. Remove from oven and place in a shallow bowl.
- Whisk together the ingredients for the sauce (sesame oil, soy sauce, maple syrup, chili garlic sauce, peanut butter) until creamy and smooth. Add 1/2 of the sauce to the tofu bowl and let marinate while you prepare the rest of the ingredients.
- Toss the broccoli with 1 teaspoon sesame or olive oil and a pinch of salt and pepper. Place in the oven and roast for 20 mins until just tender.
- Heat remaining olive or sesame oil in a large nonstick skillet over medium heat. Add tofu, in batches, along with the marinating sauce until crispy and golden browned, about 3-4 mins.
- To assemble, divide the brown rice among 4 bowls, top each bowl with 1/4 cup shredded carrots, 1/2 cup spinach leaves, 1/4th broccoli, 1/4 cup garbanzo beans and a few pieces of tofu. Drizzle with remaining peanut sauce.

Harissa Portobello Mushroom "Tacos"

Prep Time: 20 Mins - Cook Time: 10 Mins - Total Time: 30 Mins

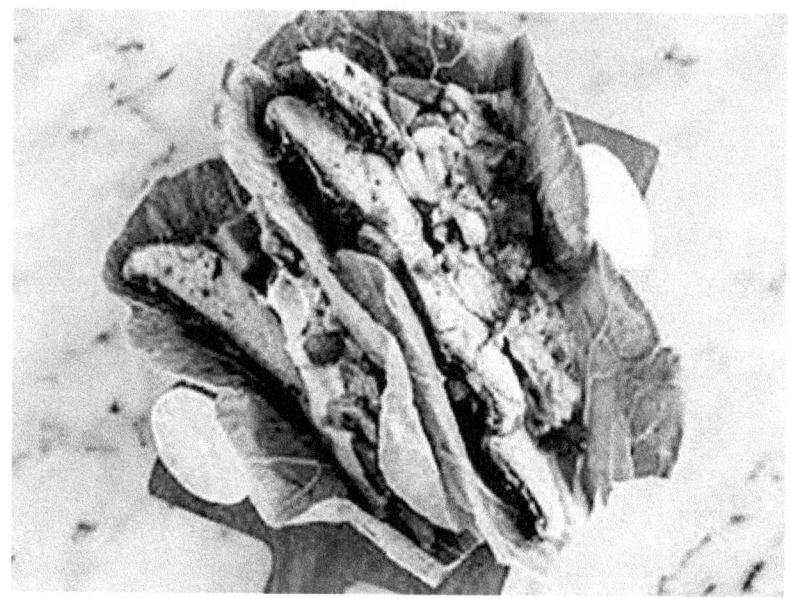

Ingredients

- Portobello Mushrooms
- 1-pound (450g) portobello mushrooms
- 1/4 cup (60g) spicy harissa, or use a mild harissa
- 3 tablespoons olive oil, divided
- 1 teaspoon ground cumin
- 1 teaspoon onion powder
- 6 collard green leaves
- Guacamole
- 2 medium ripe avocados
- 2 tablespoons chopped tomatoes

- 2 tablespoons chopped red onion
- 1 1/2 to 2 tablespoons lemon or lime juice
- pinch of salt
- 1 tablespoon chopped cilantro

Preparation

- Remove the stem of the portobellos. Rinse mushrooms and pat dry.
- Mix harissa, 1 1/2 tablespoons olive oil, cumin, and onion powder in a bowl. Brush each mushroom with the harissa mixture, making sure to cover the edges of the mushroom as well. Let mushroom marinade for 15 mins.
- While the mushrooms are marinating, prepare guacamole. Halve and pit the avocados and scoop out the flesh. Mash avocados and mix in chopped tomatoes, red onion, lemon (or lime) juice, salt, and cilantro. Set aside.
- Rinse collard greens. Chop off the tough stems and set aside.
- When the mushrooms are done marinating, heat 1 1/2 tablespoons of olive oil in a skillet or sauté pan over medium-high heat. Place the portobello mushrooms in the pan and cook for 3 mins. Flip over and cook for another 2 to 3 mins. Each side should be browned.
- Turn off the heat and let the mushrooms rest for 2 to 3 mins before slicing.
- Take a collard green leaf and fill it with a few slices of portobello. Add guacamole, chopped tomatoes, cashew cream, and cilantro to your liking.

Chapter 8

DINNER RECIPES

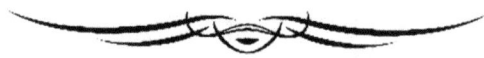

BAKED EASY CHEESY ZUCCHINI CASSEROLE

Prep Time 10 Mins - Cook Time 30 Mins - Total Time 1 Hour 25 Mins

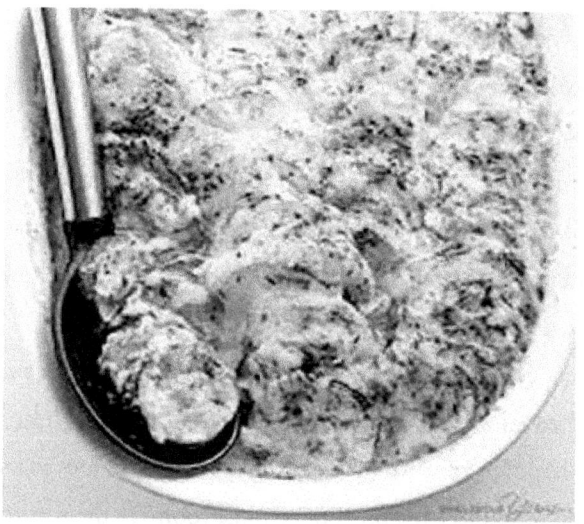

Ingredients

- » Click underlined ingredients to buy them!
- » 3 medium Zucchini (sliced in 1/4" thick slices)
- » Sea salt
- » Black pepper
- » 1 1/2 cup Swiss Gruyere shredded cheese blend (or any shredded sharp cheese; divided)

- 3 oz Brie cheese (edges cut off)
- 1/3 cup Heavy cream
- 2 tbsp Unsweetened almond milk (or any milk of choice)
- 1 tbsp Butter
- 2 cloves Garlic (minced or crushed)
- 1/2 tbsp Italian seasoning
- Wholesome Yum Keto Sweeteners

Preparation

- Toss the zucchini slices with sea salt. Place into a colander and set over the sink to drain for 45 mins. Pat dry at the end.
- Preheat the oven to 400 degrees F (204 degrees C).
- In a small 1.5 quart (1.5 L) casserole dish, arrange the zucchini slices in several overlapping rows, sprinkly very lightly with half of shredded cheese between rows. You'll use about 3/4 cup cheese total. Season lightly with black pepper. (They already have salt at this point.)
- Combine the brie, cream, milk, butter, and garlic in a small saucepan. Heat for a few mins on the stove over low to medium-low heat, stirring frequently, until the cheese melts and the mixture is smooth. If desired, add sea salt to taste. Pour the mixture evenly over the zucchini.
- Sprinkle the remaining 3/4 cup shredded cheese blend on top. Top with Italian seasoning.
- Bake for about 30-35 mins, until the cheese on top is dark golden brown and the zucchini is soft.

Vegan Coconut Curry

Time 25 Mins - Prep Time 10 Mins - Cook Time 15 Mins - Total Time 25 Mins

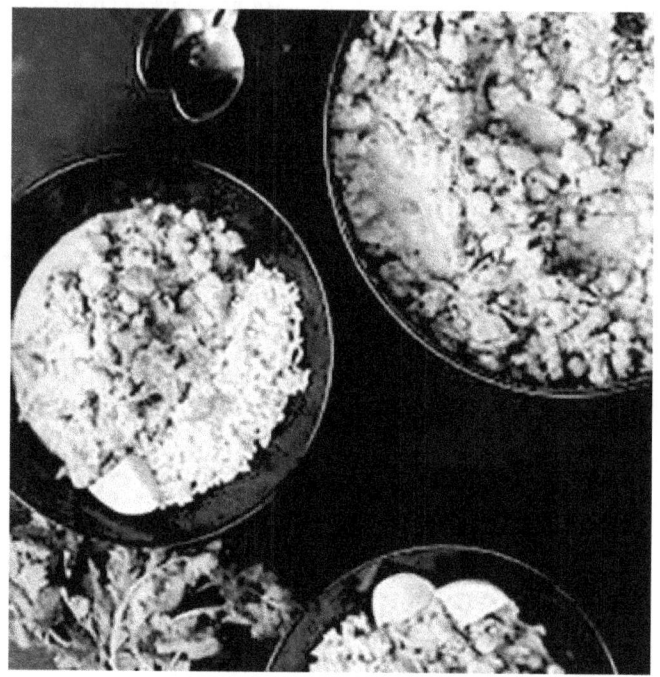

Ingredients

- 1 tbsp olive oil
- 1 cup broccoli (or use green beans)
- 1 spring onions
- 1 sweet potato
- 2 carrot
- ½ zucchini
- 2 sticks lemongrass
- 2 tsp curry powder
- 1 tbsp yellow curry paste (or red for hotter, green for hottest!)

- » 1 can coconut milk
- » 1 can chickpeas (15 oz = 435g, drained and rinsed)
- » 1 tbsp maple syrup
- » ½ tsp salt
- » 1 lemon (juiced; lime works too!)
- » Optional:
- » 1 cup basmati rice (cooked; whole grain rice is nice too)
- » ½ cup cashews (roasted; or use peanuts)

Preparation

- » If serving with rice, get that cooking now according to package Preparation .
- » Grate the sweet potato and the carrots.
- » Chop the spring onion, broccoli, and zucchini.
- » Add the olive oil to a large pan and fry all the veg on a medium heat. This needs about 5-7 mins.
- » Next, add the curry powder and curry paste, and the beaten (smack it with a heavy spoon a few times to let out the flavor) lemongrass.
- » Drain and rinse the chickpeas.
- » Stir and fry for another couple of mins then add the coconut milk, chickpeas, lemon juice, maple syrup and salt. Let it simmer for another 5 mins.
- » Alright, that's it. Take out the lemongrass. Serve with rice and top with roasted cashews or peanuts. Easy. Awesome.

One Pot Spinach Rice

Prep Time 10 Mins - Cook Time 20 Mins - Total Time 30 Mins - Servings :3

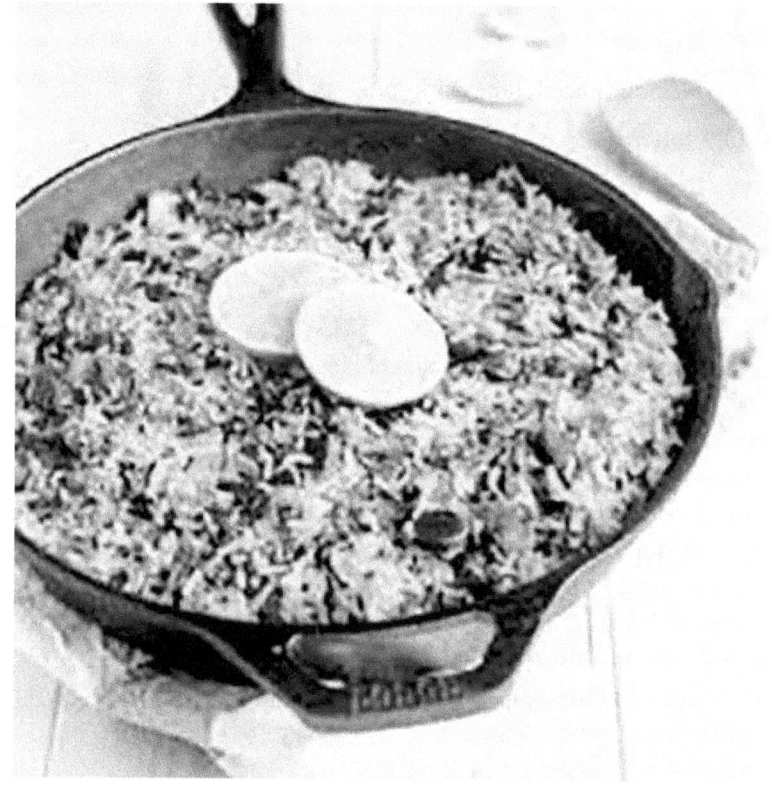

Ingredients

- » 1 cup white rice (rinsed and drained)
- » 2-3 cups fresh baby spinach
- » 2 Tomatoes diced
- » 1 medium onion diced
- » 2-3 cloves garlic minced
- » 1 cup Pinto beans canned (rinsed and drained)

- » 2 cup low sodium chicken stock (or vegetable stock or water if vegan)
- » 1 1/2 tsp curry powder
- » 1 tsp avocado oil or other cooking oil
- » salt and pepper

Preparation

- » Heat oil in a large skillet on medium heat. Add garlic and saute until fragrant for about 30 sec
- » Add onion and saute until translucent. Then add diced tomatoes and cook them until they soften for about 3-4 mins
- » Add spinach, beans, rice and cook for a couple of mins. Now add water, chicken stock or vegetable stock (if vegan) and bring the mixture to a boil
- » Season with curry powder, salt and pepper. Adjust salt and pepper according to taste
- » Simmer the rice mixture for 18-20 min (or until rice is tender) on low heat with lid on
- » Turn off the heat and serve warm to enjoy this nutritious spinach rice

Spicy Corn Chowder

Time 25 Mins - Prep Time 10 Mins - Cook Time 15 Mins - Total Time 25 Mins

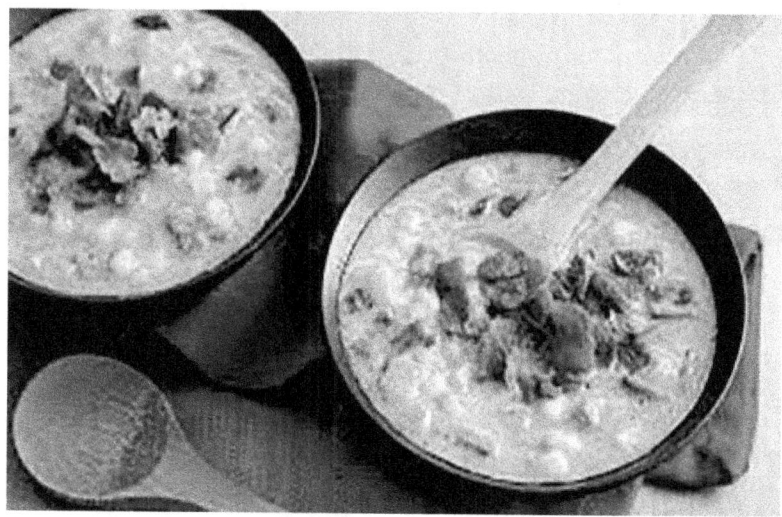

Ingredients

- 1 cup milk
- 1 cup vegetable broth
- 1 large knob butter
- ½ medium onion (diced)
- 1 tbsp all purpose flour (or rice flour to make it gluten-free)
- 1 can sweet corn (drained and rinsed)(1 can = 15 oz)
- ½ bell pepper, red (we recommend red)
- 1 chili pepper (finely chopped)
- 1 tsp cumin
- 2 tsp curry powder
- ½ cup cheddar cheese
- 2 shallots (or spring onions)

Preparation

- Heat milk and vegetable broth together in a separate pot on a low heat; make sure it doesn't boil otherwise the fat will separate itself from the milk.
- Dice up the onion, get a pot and let it simmer in the butter. Then add flour. Stir well.
- Dice up the bell pepper and add it to the pot. Throw in the corn too.
- Cut the chili pepper into small pieces and off into the pot with it.
- Now add the milk and broth mix to the pot. Stir in the cumin and curry powder too.
- Stir everything well and let it simmer for about 5 mins on a low heat.
- Finally throw in the cheddar and let it melt.
- Cut up the shallots and add them for garnish.
- That's it, enjoy your corn chowder!

Vegetarian Fajita Pasta

Prep Time: 5 mins - Cook Time: 10 mins - Total Time: 15 mins

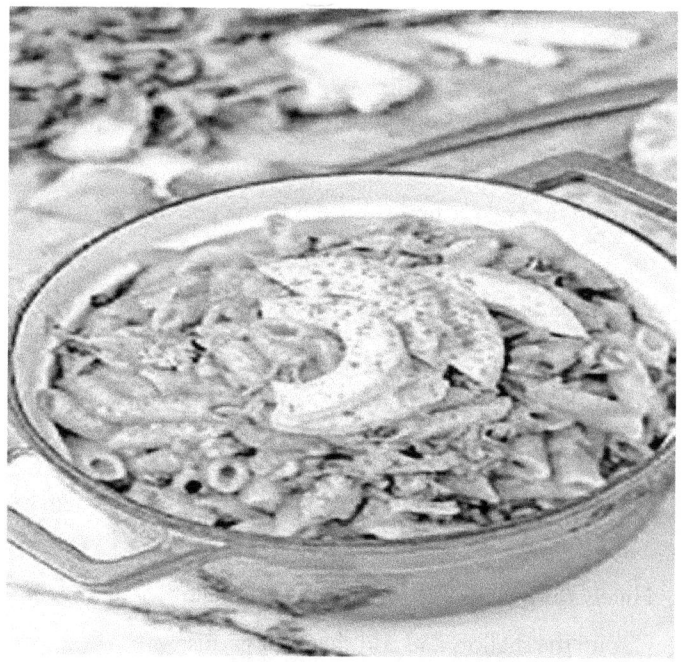

Ingredients

- 4 cups of your favorite pasta, cooked (I used gluten free)
- 2 cups Enchilada Sauce, store-bought or homemade
- 6 cloves garlic, peeled and finely chopped
- 1 cup black beans, cooked
- Taco Seasoning mix (I used 1 tsp cumin, 1 tsp chili powder, 1/2 tsp paprika)
- 1 heaping cup chopped bell peppers
- salt pepper to taste
- OPTIONAL ADD ONS:

- » 3/4 cup chopped onions
- » 1/2 cup corn
- » avocado slices

Preparation

- » Start with frying the garlic with your favorite oil. If you want to go for oil free cooking, simply use vegetable broth. If you decide to use the chopped onions now is the time to add them. Together, it will take 4 mins until all is slightly golden and brown. You will recognize a delicious smell in your kitchen.
- » Next and last add all the other ingredients (Enchilada sauce, Taco seasoning, bell pepper and your optional choices) to that pot. After 5 mins add the cooked pasta and cook for 4 mins more. Divide into bowls or plates, and serve with avocado slices on top.

Farro Salad with Green Olives, Hazelnuts and Raisins

Prep Time 10 mins - Cook Time 30 mins - Total Time 40 mins

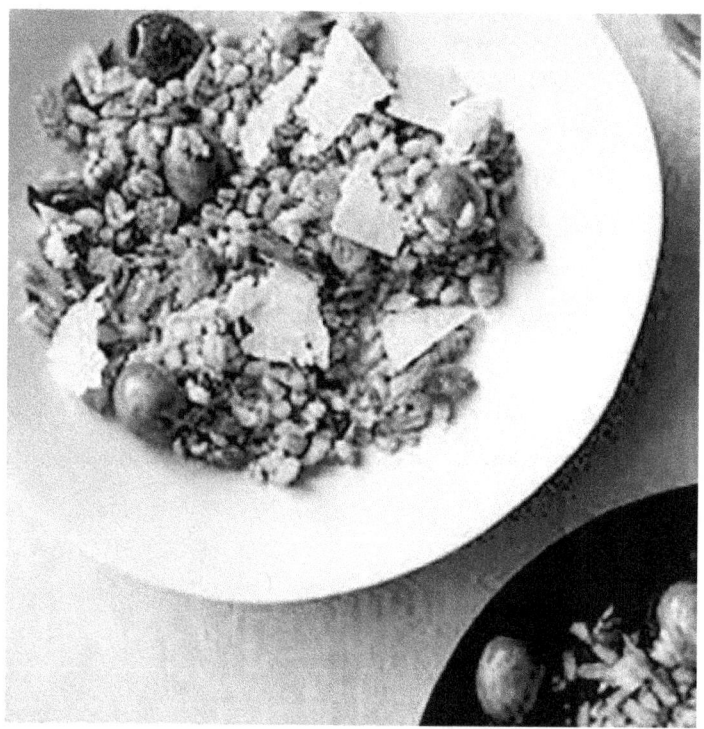

Ingredients

- » 1 1/4 cups whole farro
- » 3 cups water
- » large pinch fine-grain sea salt
- » juice of 1/2 a Meyer Lemon
- » 1 tablespoon honey
- » 1/4 cup extra-virgin olive oil

- 1 cup Castelvetrano or other buttery green olive coarsely chopped
- 1 cup toasted hazelnuts coarsely chopped
- 3 green onions roughly chopped
- 1/3 cup golden raisins look for golden Himalayan raisins – they're delicious and usually unushered
- large pinch crushed red pepper flakes
- 1 ounce shaved pecorino plus more for serving
- 1/4 cup chopped fresh Italian parsely

Preparation

- Combine farro, water, and salt in a saucepan over medium-high heat. Cover, bring to a boil, then reduce heat to a simmer. Gently simmer 30 mins, until farro is tender but not mushy. Drain excess water. Set aside to cool.
- In a large serving bowl, whisk together lemon juice, honey and olive oil. Stir in olives, hazelnuts, green onions, raisins, crushed red pepper and 1 ounce of pecorino. Add farro and toss to thoroughly combine.
- Top with parsley and several pecorino shavings; serve.

Purple Beetroot Pasta

Prep Time 10 mins - Cook Time 15 mins - Total Time 25 mins

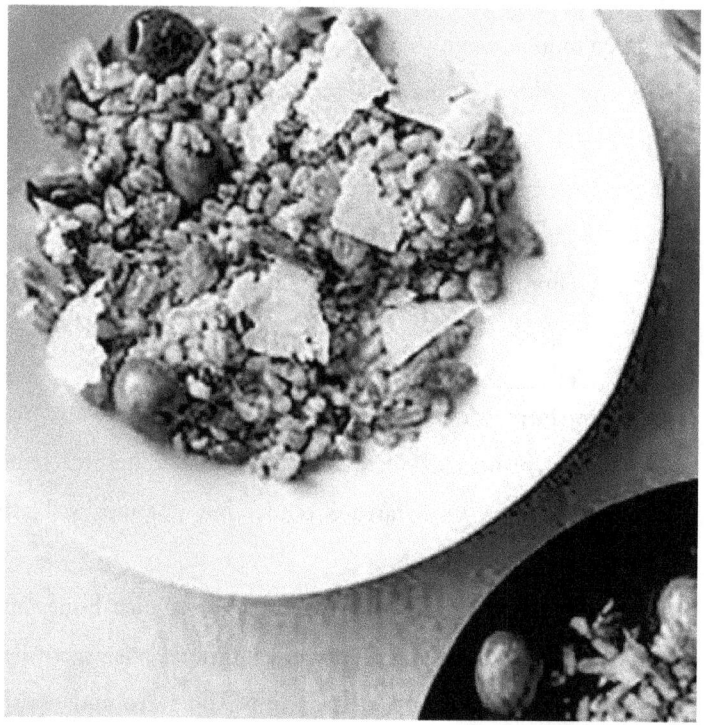

Ingredients

- 7 oz pasta
- 1 tbsp olive oil
- 1 tbsp white wine vinegar
- 1 handful walnuts
- 1 onion
- 1 clove garlic
- 2 tsp sage, fresh (dried is fine too; or rosemary)

- » 1 large beetroot, pre-cooked (or two small)
- » ½ cup feta cheese
- » 1 handful arugula/rocket (1 handful = 50g)
- » 1 lemon (sliced)
- » salt and pepper to taste
- » Optional
- » ¼ cup beetroot juice

Preparation

- » Cook pasta according to package description.
- » Roast the walnuts in a large dry pan on medium heat for a couple of mins.
- » Dice the onion and garlic.
- » Put the walnuts into a small side bowl and add the onion and garlic to the pan with olive oil on low to medium heat. After 2 mins season with sage, salt and pepper.
- » Open the packaged beetroot and pour the excess liquid into the pan. It should just be a few drops. Cut beetroot into small cubes and add it too.
- » Add the white wine vinegar to the mix.
- » Once ready, drain the pasta with a colander and collect about half a cup (100 ml) of the excess pasta water.
- » Add both the pasta and water to the pan.
- » Now it's time for the coloring, if you bought the beet juice. Add it to the mix. Give everything a good stir and let it simmer for about 6 mins and make the taste test.
- » While it's simmering, wash and roughly cut the arugula.
- » Garnish with the arugula, feta, walnuts and lemon slices.

Vegetarian Fried Rice

Prep Time 5 Mins - Cook Time 10 Mins - Total Time 15 Mins

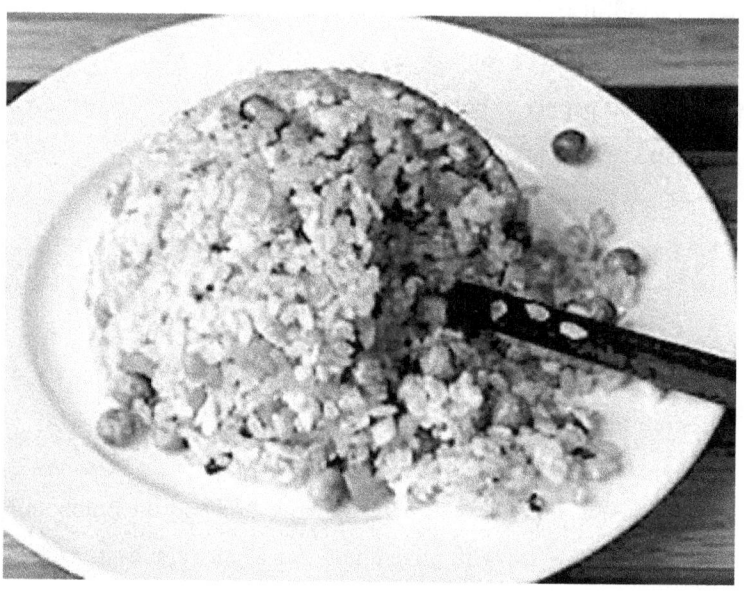

Ingredients

- For the sauce
- 2 tbsp soy sauce (dark)
- 2 tsp vinegar (eg. white wine vinegar)
- 2 tsp olive oil (or any other oil you have at hand)
- 1 tsp maple syrup
- For the fried rice
- 2 medium eggs (2 medium eggs = 1 large egg. Beaten)
- salt to taste
- 2 tbsp sesame oil (or whatever you have available)
- 3 cups rice (cooked)

- » 1 onion (or 2 spring onions, finely chopped)
- » 2 cups veggies of your choice (frozen vegetables are fine too, but make sure to thaw them before frying)

Preparation

- » In a small bowl mix together the ingredients for the sauce. Then chop your veggies into bite sized pieces.
- » Get a pan to high heat, add sesame oil and pour in the egg. While scrambling add a small dash of salt and vinegar. The egg should be done in about a mins, then set aside in a bowl.
- » Add another tbsp of oil into the pan on high heat and add the onion. Let it fry for about 30 seconds (NOTE: If you use spring onions, add them in the end instead!).
- » Now is the time to your veggies to the pan. Stir fry for 3-5 mins.
- » Reduce the heat, add the rice, sauce and your eggs. Stir well. Now you can safely add your spring onions too.

Black Bean Veggie Tacos

Prep Time: 10 Mins - Cook Time: 0 Mins - Time: 10 Mins

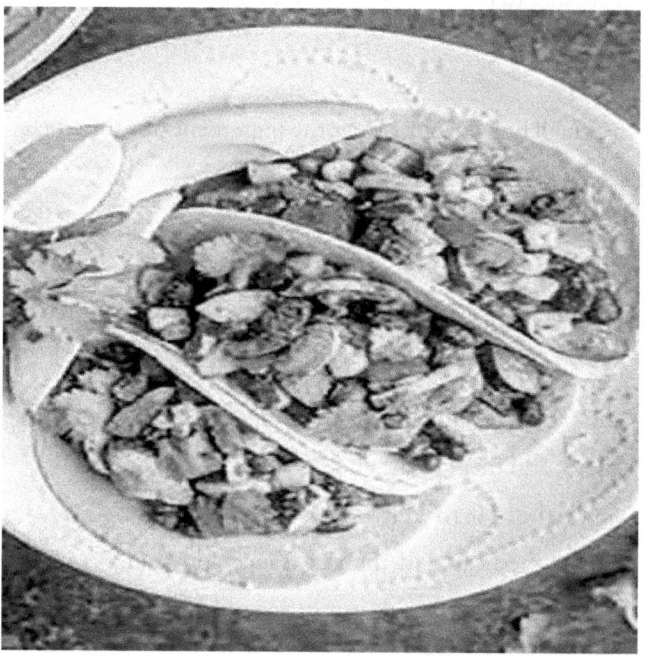

Ingredients

- » 3 taco sized tortillas corn or flour
- » 1/2 cup brown rice
- » 1/2 cup black beans
- » 1/4 whole bell pepper sliced
- » large handful shredded red cabbage
- » 1/2 cup salsa
- » 1 tablespoon favorite cheese
- » 1 tablespoon cilantro leaves
- » 1 whole lime quartered

Preparation

» Layer ingredients on top of tacos with salsa and cheese last. Enjoy

Pineapple Fried Rice

Prep Time 10 mins - Cook Time 20 mins - Total Time 30 mins

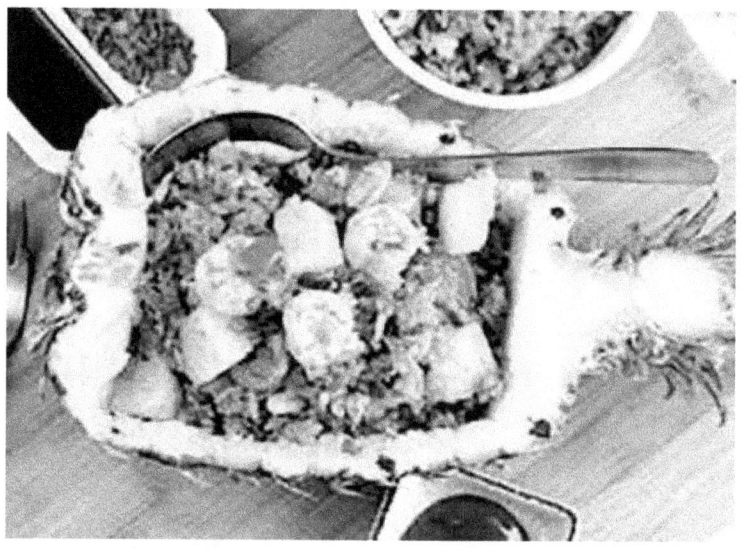

Ingredients

- 1 cup basmati rice
- 1 handful cashews
- 1 cup pineapple chunks (canned or fresh pineapple)
- 1 banana
- 1 tbsp coconut oil (other oil will do as well)
- 2 red onion
- 1 red chili pepper
- ½ cup coconut milk
- 1 bunch cilantro/coriander, fresh (parsley can be used as an alternative)
- Optional:
- ½ tsp curry powder

Preparation

- Use leftover rice or cook a new batch according to package Preparation.
- Roast the cashews on low to medium heat in a pan without fat until they start to brown, then remove them.
- Roughly chop the pineapple and banana. Dice up the red onion and chilli.
- Fry the pineapple cubes in the pan with a little oil. Add the diced onion. When these are glazed, add chili and banana cubes. After 3-4 mins pour everything in a small bowl.
- Roughly clean pan, fry rice in a little oil for 3-5 mins.
- When the rice has been roasted, stir in the coconut milk.
- Now it's time to mix the cashew nuts and pineapple banana sauce.
- Finish of with some salt and pepper and if you like, a dash of curry powder.
- Ready to serve. Don't forget to garnish with cilantro!

CRUSTLESS SPINACH CHEESE PIE

Prep Time 2 Mins - Cook Time 30 Mins - Total Time 32 Mins

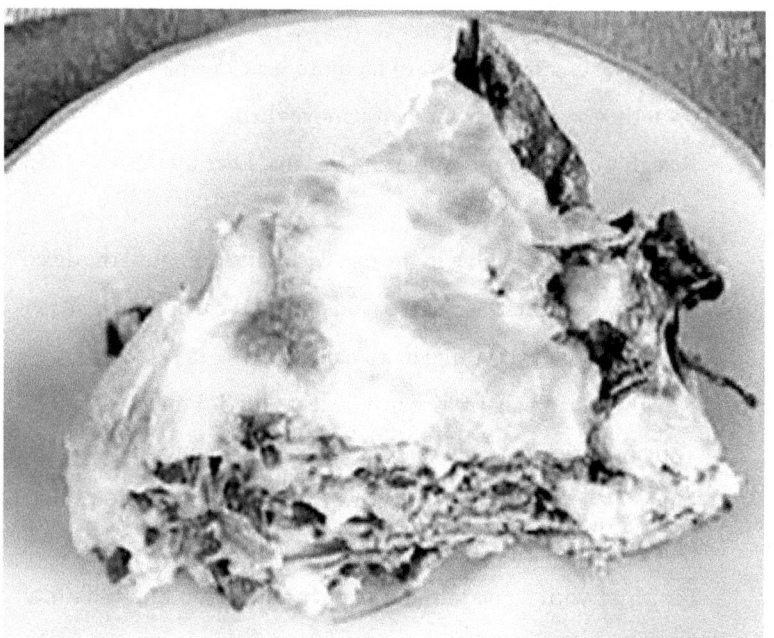

Ingredients

- » 10 ounces frozen spinach thawed, squeezed and drained (or use wilted down fresh)
- » 5 eggs beaten
- » 2 1/2 cups cheese any kind (I used a fiesta blend)
- » 1 teaspoon dried minced onion
- » 1/4 teaspoon garlic powder
- » salt and pepper to taste

Preparation

- Grease a 9-inch pie pan.
- Combine all ingredients and pour into prepared pan.
- Bake at 375 degrees F for about 30 mins or until edges start to brown.

Cauliflower Alfredo with Peas

Prep Time 20 Min - Cook Time 25 Min

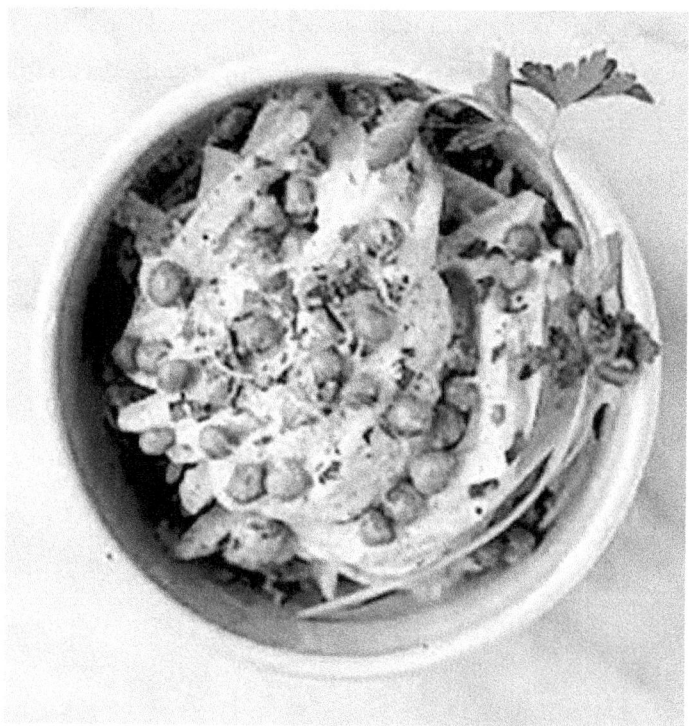

Ingredients

- » 3 cloves garlic, roughly chopped
- » 1 large head of cauliflower, stem and leaves removed, roughly chopped
- » 1 cup chicken or vegetable broth (or water, but broth will taste better)
- » 1/2 tsp salt
- » 2 tbsp unsalted butter

- » 1/2-1 cup whole milk
- » 1/4-1/2 cup finely grated parmesan cheese, plus more for serving
- » 1 lb (454 grams) of fettuccine
- » 1 cup frozen, canned, or fresh peas
- » fresh ground pepper, to taste
- » 1 tsp chopped fresh parsley to garnish, optional

Preparation

- » Place garlic, cauliflower, and chicken broth in a large saucepan with a lid. Bring to a boil, reduce heat to medium-low and cook for 8-10 mins (or until cauliflower is tender and soft).
- » Carefully transfer contents of saucepan to a blender or a food processor (blend will result in a smoother consistency).
- » Add salt, butter, 1/2 cup milk, and parmesan cheese. Blend on high until desired consistency is reached (I prefer a smooth texture). Add in remaining 1/2 cup milk if sauce is too thick. Taste and season with more salt if required.
- » Meanwhile, cook fettuccine as per package Preparation, adding peas with 1 mins left in the cooking time. Drain pasta and peas. Toss with cauliflower alfredo sauce.
- » Garnish with more parmesan and/or chopped fresh parsley if desired.

Spicy Black Bean Soup

Prep Time 7 Mins - Cook Time 13 Mins - Total Time 20 Mins

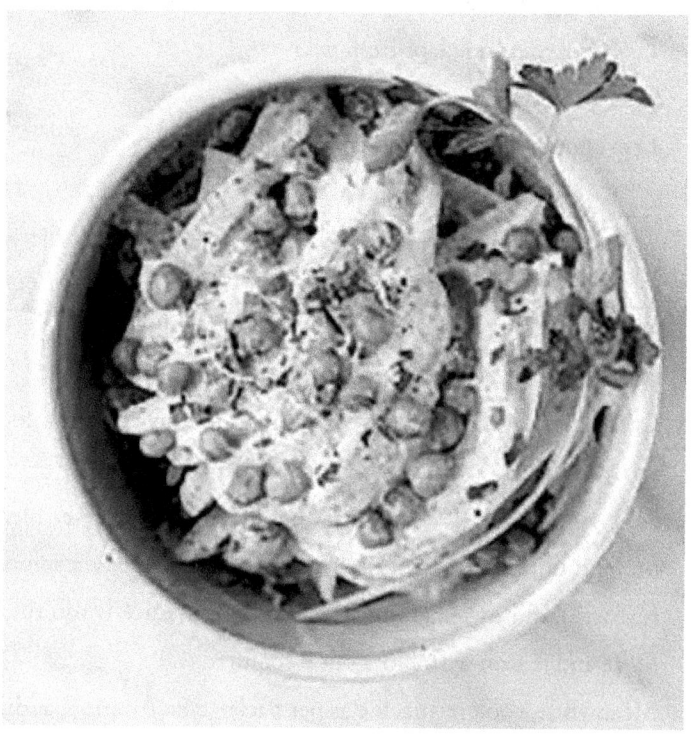

Ingredients

- 1 tbsp olive oil
- ½ onion
- 2 cloves garlic
- 1 bell pepper, red
- 1 can black beans (1 can = 15.5oz)
- 250 ml vegetable broth
- ⅛ cup cilantro/coriander, fresh

- » 1.5 tsp cumin
- » ¼ tsp red pepper flakes (be careful not to make it too hot!!)
- » 1 tbsp balsamic vinegar
- » ½ avocado
- » Optional
- » 2 tortillas
- » 1 slice cheddar cheese (only for those who are not vegan)

Preparation

- » Get a pot and add one tbsp of olive oil.
- » Finely dice up the onion and mince the garlic. Throw both in the pot and let it simmer on low heat.
- » In the meantime cut the bell pepper into small pieces and add them to the pot.
- » Rinse and drain the can of black beans.
- » Squash a few of them with a fork or your hands to give the soup a creamy touch, then throw them into the pot with a bit of love.
- » Add the vegetable broth to the mix.
- » Chop the cilantro and add it to the soup (holding a bit in reserve for garnish).
- » Now pimp it up with the cumin, red pepper flakes and balsamic vinegar.
- » Let the soup simmer for about 10 mins.
- » In the meantime prepare some avocado slices and heat up the tortillas.
- » If you want to be naughty, finish off the soup with a slice of cheddar.

- » Taste test – adjust the seasoning, if necessary.
- » Soups on! Garnish the bowl with a little extra cilantro, avocado and you're ready to roll.

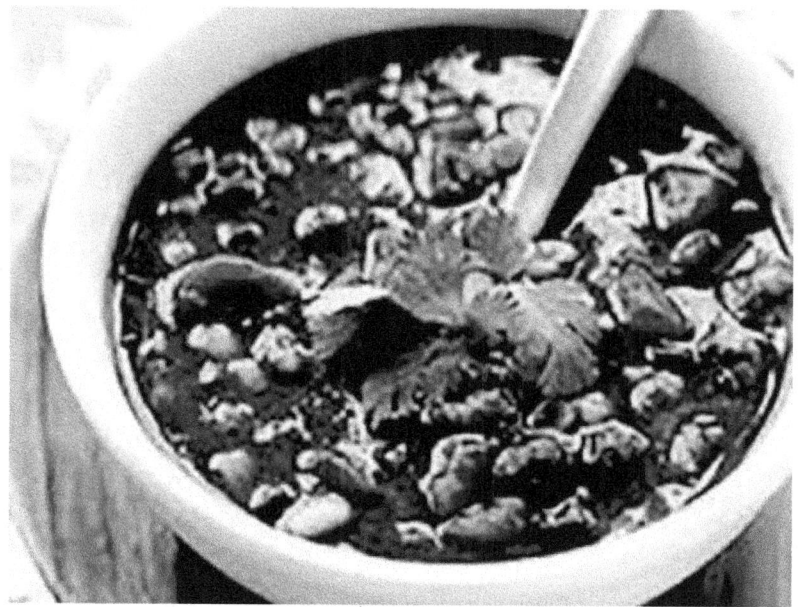

DINNER RECIPES

Crispy Tortilla Pizza

Prep Time 10 Mins - Cook Time 15 Mins - Total Time 25 Mins

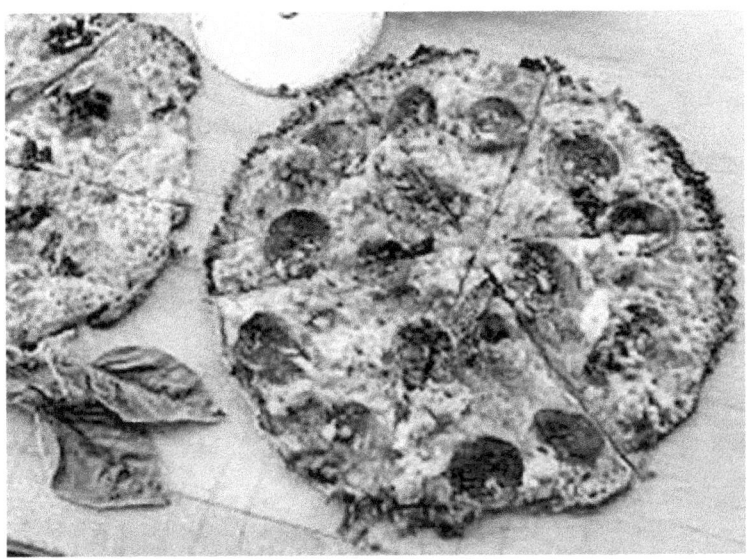

Ingredients

- » 4 tortillas (whole wheat ideally)
- » 1 tomato puree
- » 1 ball mozzarella cheese (feta or most other cheeses work fine)
- » 1 handful olives
- » 1 white or red onion
- » 1 chilli / jalapeño
- » 4 small tomato
- » ½ bell pepper, red (your fave colour)
- » ½ cup basil, fresh (dried is fine but use much less)
- » Optional
- » ½ can sweet corn (drained and rinsed) (½ can = 7.5 oz)

Preparation

- » Spread the tomato puree over each tortilla.
- » Lob on the basil.
- » Slice the cheese into thin layers and add to tortillas.
- » Chop the veggies into small pieces then place evenly on tortillas
- » Cook in the oven for 10-15 mins at 180°C (360°F) - don't let the tortillas burn!
- » Munch.

Roasted Chiles Rellenos with Black Beans

Prep Time: 20 - Cook Time: 60 - Total Time: 1 Hour 20

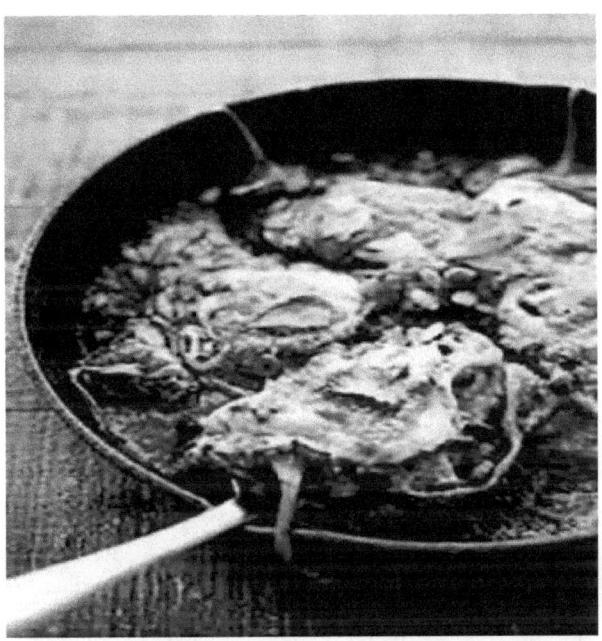

Ingredients

- 4–6 extra-large poblano peppers, leave whole with stems on. (see notes)
- 6 ripe, medium tomatoes, (roma, or vine-ripened)
- 6 fat garlic cloves
- one large onion, sliced into ½ inch wedges or slices
- 2 small jalapeños
- 2 tablespoons olive oil
- FILLING

- 14 ounce can black beans, drained and rinsed -seasoned (see notes) or Cuban Style are nice
- 6 ounces grated jack cheese or Mexican queso fresco (or 1 cup vegan Herbed Tofu Ricotta)
- SAUCE ADDITIONS:
- 2 teaspoons cumin
- 1 teaspoon coriander
- 1 teaspoon chili powder
- 1 teaspoon dried oregano
- 1 teaspoon salt
- 1 tablespoon tomato paste (optional, but good)
- ¼ cup fresh cilantro plus more for garnish
- 1/4–1/2 cup water or broth (to the desired consistency)
- Serve with cilantro lime rice, sour cream, hot sauce, avocado, toasted pumpkin seeds, cilantro

Preparation

- Preheat oven to 45oF Cut the tomatoes in half and arrange them on the sheet pan. Add the sliced onions to sheet pan, along with the whole garlic cloves, halved jalapeños and whole poblano peppers, making sure they are not overcrowded. You may need to use two sheet pans. (You can also char the peppers on a gas burner, see notes) Drizzle all with olive oil, sprinkle with salt and pepper and place on the middle rack and check after 15 mins. (If your oven runs hot, you could turn it down to 425 if needed.) If the peppers are tender remove them (pasilla peppers will cook much faster than poblanos- please see notes) and check the garlic, removing it if tender. Otherwise continue roasting with the tomatoes and onions another 15-20 mins, until peppers and onions are tender and tomatoes are juicy.

- » In the meantime make the filling: Mix the canned beans (drained, rinsed) with the cheese. OR If going vegan, mix the beans with 1 cup of vegan herbed tofu ricotta. Season the mixture with salt and pepper. If using plain black beans, add a teaspoon of cumin and chili powder.
- » When the poblanos are just tender, take the sheet pan out of the oven (leave the oven on) and let it cool.
- » Add ⅓ of the onions, chopping them up, and add into the filling mixture and stir.
- » Blend up the Roasted Ranchos Sauce: Place the remaining onions into a blender along with the tomatoes, pan juices, jalapeño, garlic, cumin, coriander, chili powder, oregano, salt, tomato paste and fresh cilantro, adding a little water (or broth if needed) to thin it out, and blend until smooth. Set aside.
- » STUFF POBLANOS: Carefully cut a slit in the poblano peppers from stem to pointy end and using your fingers, gently remove seeds while rinsing them under cold running water. If the thin skins slip off, let them, but don't worry about actively peeling them, especially poblanos – their skins are quite thin -leaving some of the skin on is perfectly fine. Pasillo peppers have thick skin and should be peeled. In a large greased baking dish (or oven-proof skillet) pour a little of the roasted tomato ranchero sauce to coat the bottom (use about half the sauce). Place the peppers over top of the sauce, slit side up, then spoon

the black bean filling into each one. Pour the rest of the flavorful ranchero sauce over top. At this point, you could add more shredded cheese to the top, or leave it off.

- Cover with foil and bake 20-25 mins in a 425F oven- or until the filling is warm and melty, uncover and bake 5 more mins.
- Garnish with cilantro leaves, toasted pumpkin seeds and sour cream if you like

DINNER RECIPES

Vegetarian Enchiladas

Prep Time: 40 - Cook Time: 25 - Total Time: 1 Hour 5 Mins

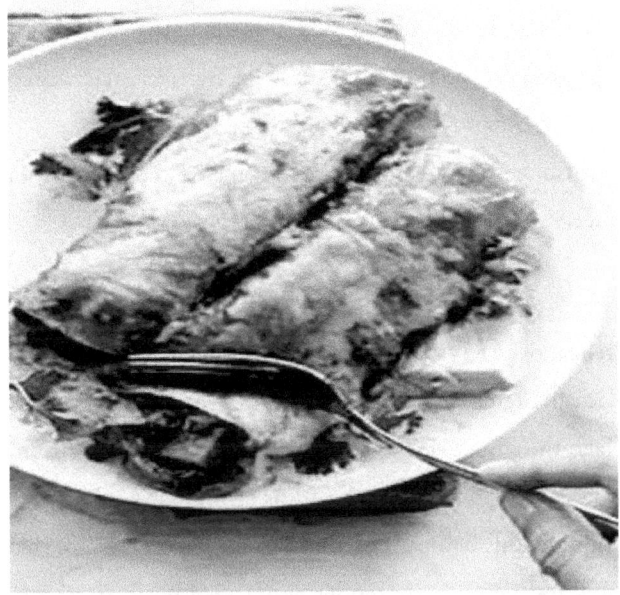

Ingredients

- 1–2 tablespoons olive oil
- 1 onion diced
- 4 garlic cloves, rough chopped
- 1 red bell pepper diced
- 1 small yam, diced small (or sub zucchini)
- 1/2 teaspoon salt
- 1 ear of corn, kernels cut off (about 1 cup) or sub other veggies!
- teaspoon cumin
- 1 teaspoon coriander
- 1 teaspoon dried oregano

- » 14 ounce can black beans rinsed, drained
- » 1/4 cup chopped cilantro (optional)
- » cups homemade enchilada sauce (or store-bought)
- » 8 x 8-inch whole wheat tortillas (or sub corn)
- » cups grated cheese (8-10 ounces pepper jack, Mexican blend, cheddar, Mozzarella) or sub vegan cheese!
- » Garnishes: sour cream, avocado, pickled red onions and hot sauce.

Preparation

- » Preheat oven to 400 F If making the homemade enchilada sauce, place all ingredients in a blender and blend until smooth.
- » Make the filling: Heat oil in a large skillet over medium-high heat. Add onion and stir 2-3 mins until fragrant. Lower heat to medium adds bell pepper, yams, garlic and salt. Sauté this until yams and peppers are tender about -7-9 mins. If mixture gets dry, add a splash of water, lower heat and cover and gently steam until yams are fork-tender. Fold in the fresh corn and cumin, coriander and oregano. Saute 3 more mins. Remove from heat. Add the black beans, taste for salt, adding more if you like. Stir in half the cilantro.
- » Grease a 9 x 13 baking dish. Pour 1/2 cup of the enchilada sauce and spreading around so the bottom of the pan is nicely coated.
- » Assemble your Enchiladas: Place 1/2 cup filling down the center of the tortilla add 2-3 tablespoons grated cheese over top and wrap it up tightly. Place enchilada seam side down over the sauce. Repeat with the remaining 7 tortillas nestling them side by side.

Pour the remaining Enchilada Sauce over the enchiladas, leaving the edges exposed if you like (for crispy edges). Sprinkle with remaining cup of cheese.

- Place in the hot oven, foiled for 20 mins then uncover for the last 6-10 mins until cheese is nice and melty. Let stand 10-15 mins before serving (tented with foil). Scatter the remaining chopped cilantro over the enchiladas. Serve with sour cream and hot sauce. Serve

Mushroom Wellington with Rosemary and Pecans

Prep Time: 45 - Cook Time: 35 - Total Time: 1 hour 20 mins

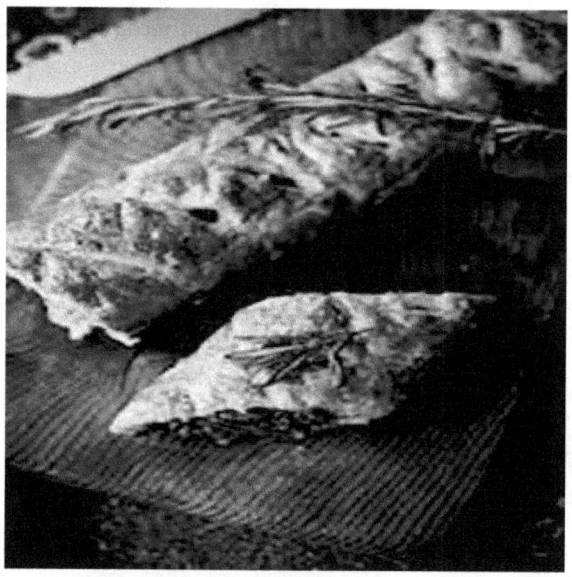

Ingredients

- » 2 sheets vegan puff pastry, thawed in the fridge overnight.
- » 2 tablespoons olive oil (or butter)
- » 2 pounds mushrooms, sliced, stems OK (except Shiitake stems)
- » 1 large onion, diced
- » 4–6 fat garlic cloves, rough chopped
- » 1 tablespoon chopped fresh rosemary (or sage, or thyme)
- » 1 teaspoon kosher salt
- » 1/4 cup sherry wine (not sherry vinegar) marsala wine, ruby port (or red wine or white wine) – or leave it out! see notes.

- 1 teaspoon balsamic vinegar
- 1 cup chopped, toasted pecans (or feel free to sub hazelnuts or walnuts)
- ½ teaspoon pepper
- 2 teaspoons truffle oil (optional)
- OPTIONS -if you want to add cheese, add ½ – 1 cup grated pecorino, gruyere, goat cheese or cream cheese
- "Egg" wash – use nut milk, cream or melted coconut oil to brush on the pastry. If not worried about it being vegan, whisk an egg with a tablespoon of water.

Preparation

- Make sure your puff pastry is thawed before you start.
- Preheat oven to 400F
- Heat oil in an extra-large skillet or dutch oven, over medium-high heat. Add mushrooms, onions, garlic, salt and rosemary and saute, stirring often, until mushrooms release all their liquid. Turn heat down to medium, and continue sauteing until all the liquid has evaporated, be patient, this will take a little time! Once the mushrooms are relatively dry in the pan, splash with the sherry wine and balsamic vinegar and again, sauté on medium heat until all the liquid has cooked off. This is important- you absolutely do not want a watery filling (it will turn into a mess!). Add the toasted chopped pecans, pepper, truffle oil. Taste, adjust salt to your liking. At this point, you could fold in some cheese if you like.

- Let the filling cool 15-20 mins (you could make the filling a day ahead and refrigerate).
- Fill Pastry: When the filling is at room temp, unroll the puff pastry onto a parchment-lined baking sheet. Place half the filling in a mound along the center (see photo) and working quickly, roll the pastry up, and over, seam side down. Fill and roll the second sheet.
- Brush with the egg or eggless wash.
- Score the pastry using a razor blade or sharp knife with your choice of design – cross-hatch, herringbone, leafy vine or just simple diagonal slits.
- Bake: Place sheet pan on the middle rack in the oven for 35 mins, checking at 20 mins, and rotating pan for even browning if necessary. Let the pastry bake until it is a really deep golden color – to ensure it's done and flaky all the way through. You may need to add 5 more mins depending on your oven. Convection will help if you have this setting (use it for the last 10 mins) Please, let's not have any pale pastries!!! Nice and golden!
- Cool for 5-10 mins before cutting and serving. Garnish with Rosemary Sprigs. It's OK to serve at room temp, but warm is best.

Roasted Cauliflower Enchiladas

Prep Time: 10 Mins - Cook Time: 25 Mins - Total Time: 35 Mins

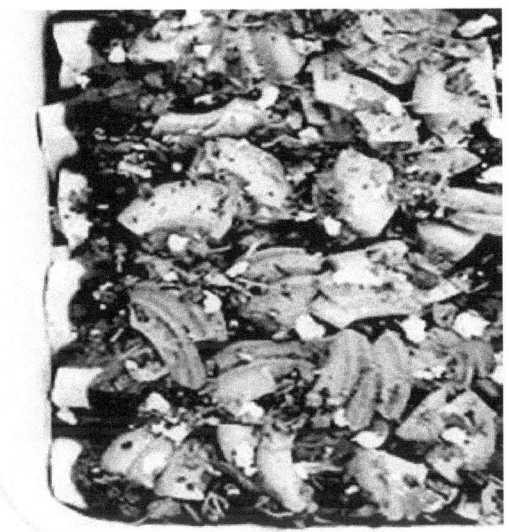

Ingredients

- 1 medium head of cauliflower, cut into florets
- 2 tablespoons olive oil
- 1 teaspoon fine sea salt
- 1/2 teaspoon freshly-cracked black pepper
- 1/4 teaspoon garlic powder

Preparation

- » Heat oven to 400°F. Line a rimmed baking sheet with parchment paper* or grease with cooking spray.
- » Spread the cauliflower out evenly on the baking sheet. Then drizzle with the olive oil, and sprinkle evenly with the salt, pepper and garlic powder. Toss gently to evenly coat the cauliflower.
- » Bake for 25-30 mins, until soft and lightly golden.
- » Serve immediately.

DINNER RECIPES

Black Bean Chili!

Prep Time: 10 Mins - Cook Time: 40 Mins - Total Time: 50 Mins

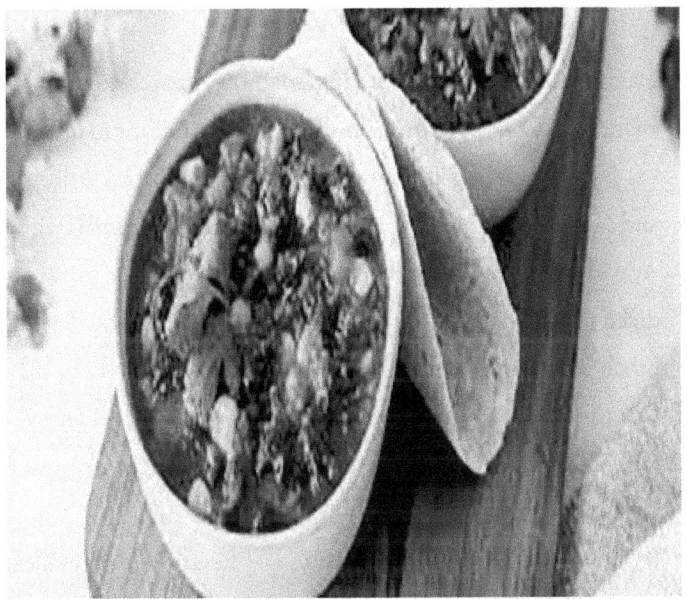

Ingredients

- 1 pound dry black beans, rinsed and picked over
- 1 medium white onion, peeled and diced
- 6 cloves garlic, peeled and minced
- 6–8 cups vegetable stock (or water*)
- 2 cups (16 ounces) salsa Verde, homemade or store-bought
- 1 (15-ounce) can fire-roasted diced tomatoes
- 1 (12-ounce) jar roasted red peppers, drained and diced
- 1 tablespoon ground cumin
- 2 teaspoons chipotle chili powder**
- salt and pepper, to taste

- » toppings: diced avocado, chopped fresh cilantro, diced red onion, shredded cheese, sliced jalapeños or serrano's

Preparation

- » Heat 1 tablespoon oil (extra ingredient for stovetop version) in a large stockpot over medium-high heat. Add onion and sauté for 5 mins, stirring occasionally, until translucent. Add garlic and sauté for 1-2 more mins, stirring occasionally, until fragrant.
- » Add in beans (pre-soaked overnight***) 6 cups stock, salsa verde, diced tomatoes, roasted red peppers, cumin, chili powder, and a pinch of salt and pepper. Stir to combine.
- » Continue cooking until the soup reaches a simmer. Then reduce heat to medium-low, cover, and cook for 45 mins, or until the beans are completely tender, stirring occasionally.
- » If you would like a brothier soup, feel free to add in 1-2 extra cups of vegetable stock. (If not, leave the soup as-is.) Taste, and season with extra salt and pepper as needed.
- » Serve immediately, garnished with lots of your favorite toppings. Or transfer to sealed containers and refrigerate for up to 3 days, or freeze for up to 3 month

Cold Sesame Peanut Noodles

Prep Time: 25 Mins - Cook Time: 5 Mins - Total Time: 30 Mins

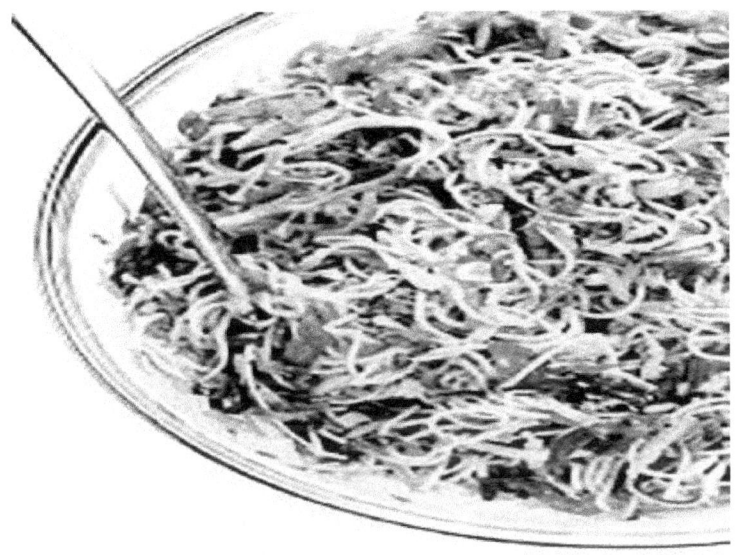

Ingredients

- NOODLE INGREDIENTS:
- 8 ounces Chinese egg noodles (or your preferred kind of noodle[1])
- 2 large carrots, grated[2] or diced
- 1 English cucumber, grated or diced
- half of a small red cabbage, finely chopped
- 2/3 cup chopped fresh cilantro
- 1/2 cup thinly-sliced green onions
- toppings: chopped peanuts, toasted sesame seeds, extra cilantro, lime wedges
- SESAME PEANUT SAUCE INGREDIENTS:

- » 1/4 cup natural peanut butter
- » 1/4 cup freshly-squeezed lime juice
- » 2–3 tablespoons low-sodium soy sauce
- » 2 tablespoons rice vinegar
- » 1 tablespoon honey or maple syrup (optional)
- » 1 tablespoon toasted sesame oil
- » 1/2 teaspoon each: garlic powder, ground ginger, black pepper, crushed red pepper flakes

Preparation

- » Cook the noodles al dente according to package Preparation. Drain, then rinse with cold water in a colander until the noodles are chilled.
- » Meanwhile, make your sesame peanut sauce. Whisk all ingredients together in a bowl until combined. Taste and add extra soy sauce, if needed. Also, if the sauce seems too thick (it should be thin enough to drizzle), whisk in a tablespoon or two of water.
- » Add noodles, carrots, cucumber, cabbage, cilantro, green onions and sesame peanut sauce to a large mixing bowl. Toss until evenly combined.
- » Serve cold, topped with your desired garnishes. Or transfer to a sealed container and refrigerate for up to 4 days.

Chapter 9

Dessert Based Diet Recipes

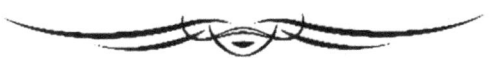

Baked Apple Pie Taquitos with Cinnamon

Total Time: 1 hours - Hands-on Time: 20 mins

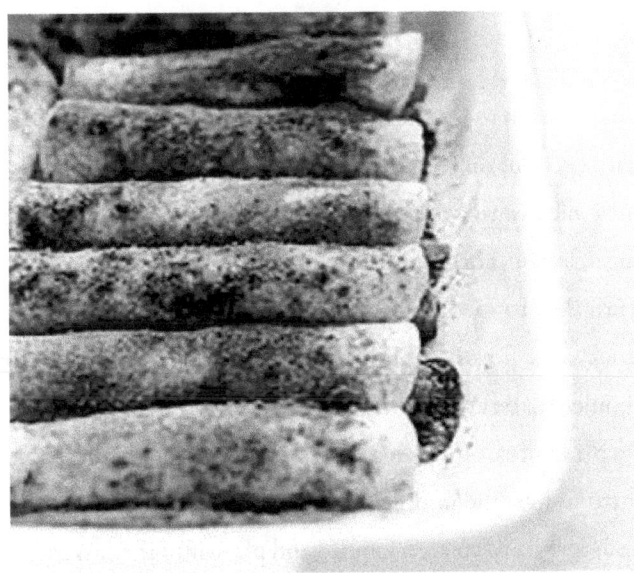

Ingredients

- » 3 teaspoons Simply Organic Cinnamon 2.45 oz.
- » 1/2 teaspoon Simply Organic Nutmeg Ground 2.30 oz.
- » 16 4-inch flour tortillas

- 4 cups apple, peeled and finely diced
- 2 tablespoons white whole wheat flour
- 1/4 cup + 3 teaspoons coconut sugar
- Squeeze of lemon
- 1 tablespoon coconut oil
- 1/2 cup + 2 tablespoons water
- 8 Medrol dates, pitted
- Pinch of salt
- add ingredients to cart
- add ingredients to shopping list

Preparation

- Preheat oven to 350 degrees. Spray a 9-by-12-inch casserole dish with coconut oil cooking spray and set aside.
- In a medium-size saucepan, combine apples, flour, coconut sugar, lemon, coconut oil, water, cinnamon and nutmeg.
- Turn heat to medium-high and let mixture cook down until a thick sauce forms (about 5 to 7 mins), stirring often. The apples should still be a bit crunchy at this point.
- Prep taquitos by placing 1 to 2 tablespoons of the apple pie mixture into the middle of each 4-inch tortilla. Tightly roll up each tortilla to create a taquito and place into the casserole dish.
- In a small bowl, mix together coconut sugar and cinnamon.
- Generously spray tops of taquitos with coconut oil cooking spray or rub with coconut oil. Sprinkle tops of taquitos with cinnamon sugar. Spray again with cooking spray.
- Bake for 35 to 40 mins.

- Meanwhile, into a high-speed food processor combine dates, water and salt. Process on high until a paste forms. Add more water, if needed.
- Let taquitos cool and serve with date caramel and ice cream.

Baked Apple with Cinnamon Goat Cheese

Total Time: 45 Mins - Hands-On Time: 10 Mins

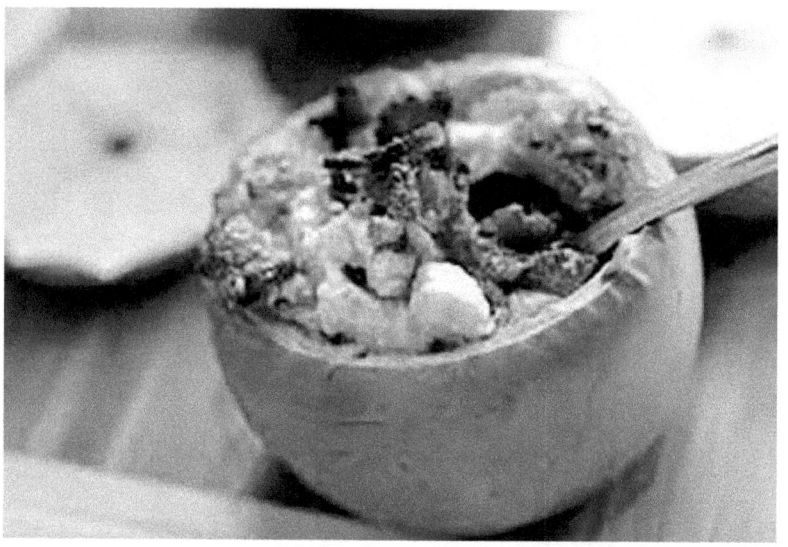

Ingredients

- 1 teaspoon Simply Organic Spice Right Cinnamon Sugar Trio 3.1 oz.
- 1 Medium-large apple (Granny Smith, Honeycrisp, Braeburn or your favorite baking apple)
- 1-ounce Plain goat cheese (chèvre variety), slightly softened
- 1 Large handful raisins (golden or regular)
- 1 Small handful walnut pieces
- add ingredients to cart
- add ingredients to shopping list

Preparation

- Heat oven to 350 degrees.
- Using a paring knife or an apple corer, carefully core the apple, leaving at least 1 1/2 inches of apple intact on the bottom. Cut around the top of the apple, so the hole is wider at the top of the apple.
- In a small bowl, combine goat cheese, raisins and cinnamon sugar trio. Fill the cavity of the apple with the goat cheese mixture, pushing it down just far enough so the mixture sits right at the top.
- In a small dish or ramekin (one that is deep enough so it props up the apple so it doesn't collapse), place the apple and bake for 30 to 35 mins, until goat cheese is starting to melt and apple is getting soft.
- Top with walnuts and a sprinkling of cinnamon sugar trio and bake for another 7 to 10 mins, until apple is just about to collapse and walnuts are toasted, being careful not to over-bake. Let cool 3 to 5 mins. Serve warm.
- To increase sweetness, substitute mascarpone goat cheese for the chèvre

Carrot Cake Muffins with Coconut Oil and Nutmeg

Total Time: 30 Mins

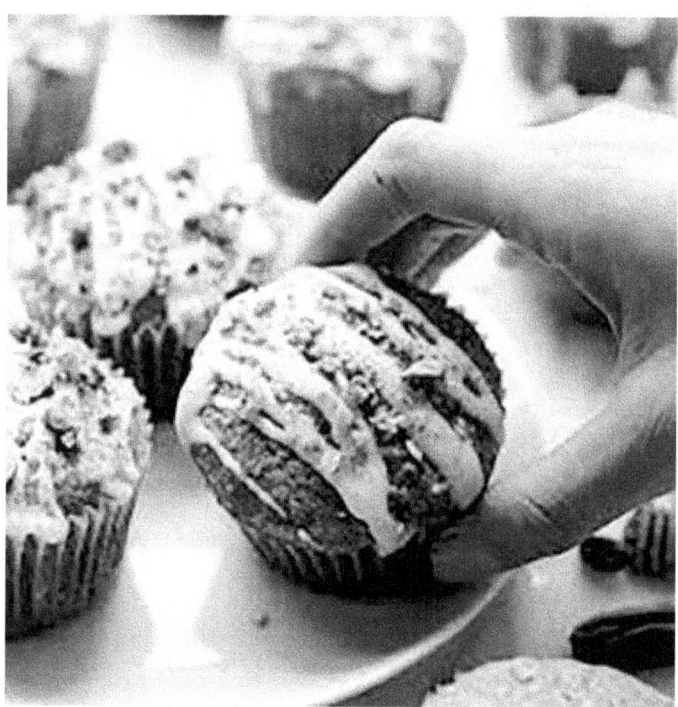

Ingredients

- 1 1/2 teaspoons Simply Organic Cinnamon 2.45 oz.
- 1/2 teaspoon Simply Organic Ginger Root Ground 1.64 oz.
- 1/2 teaspoon Simply Organic Nutmeg Ground 2.30 oz.
- 1 teaspoon Simply Organic Pure Vanilla Extract 2 fl. oz.
- 1 cup grated carrots, squeezed and packed
- 3/4 cup white whole wheat flour
- 3/4 cup all-purpose baking flour

- 1/2 cup organic cane sugar
- 1 teaspoon baking powder
- 1 teaspoon baking soda
- 1/3 cup pecans, chopped
- 1/4 cup raisins
- 1/8 teaspoon sea salt
- 2 eggs, large (separated)
- 1/4 cup plain Greek yogurt
- 1/3 cup 100% pure maple syrup
- 1 cup almond milk, unsweetened
- 1/4 cup coconut oil, partially melted
- 3/4 cup powdered sugar
- 2 tablespoons water
- add ingredients to cart
- add ingredients to shopping list

Preparation

- Preheat oven to 350 degrees.
- Place 16 muffin liners into muffin tin and set aside.
- In a medium size bowl, combine dry ingredients. Stir until well mixed, then set aside.
- In large bowl, combine egg yolks (place the egg whites into a smaller separate bowl), Greek yogurt, vanilla, maple syrup and almond milk. Using a hand mixer, mix until well combined.
- Slowly add wet ingredients into dry ingredients and mix. Then add carrots and partially melted coconut oil. Mix and set aside.

- In a separate bowl, whip the egg whites until they form peaks. Then, gently fold egg whites into batter.
- Fill muffin liners 3/4 full with batter.
- Place muffin tins into oven on middle rack for 19 to 21 mins or until a toothpick comes out clean after insertion into a muffin.
- Cool muffins for at least 30 mins before topping with icing
- To make icing, mix together powdered sugar and water. Drizzle icing over top of muffins, add chopped pecans and enjoy

Chocolate Chunk Banana Nice Cream with Cinnamon

Total Time: 5 Mins - Hands-On Time: 5 Mins

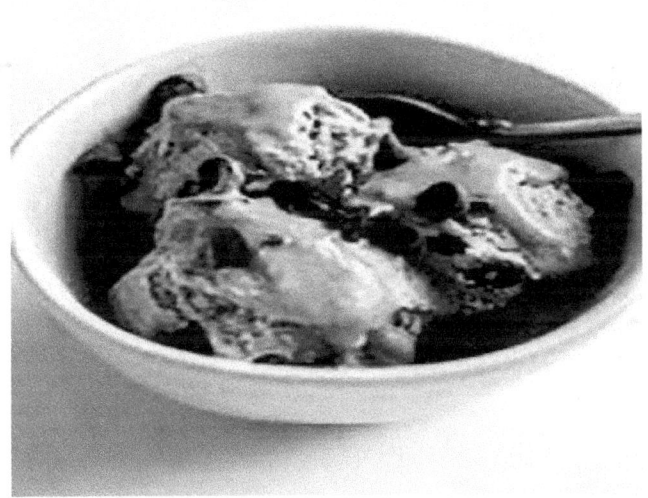

Ingredients

- » 1/2 teaspoon Simply Organic Ground Ceylon Cinnamon 2.08 oz.
- » 1 teaspoon Simply Organic Pure Vanilla Extract 2 fl. oz.
- » 4 medium ripe bananas, sliced and frozen 4 hours or overnight
- » 1 tablespoon almond (or other non-dairy) milk
- » 1/4 cup dark chocolate chips
- » add ingredients to cart
- » add ingredients to shopping list

Preparation

- In a food processor, combine frozen bananas, milk, cinnamon and vanilla. Blend until smooth. If bananas don't puree well, add a little more almond milk and continue to process.
- Add chocolate chips and pulse until chopped.
- serve immediately.

Clementine Upside Down Cupcakes

Total Time: 45 Mins - Hands-On Time: 20 Mins

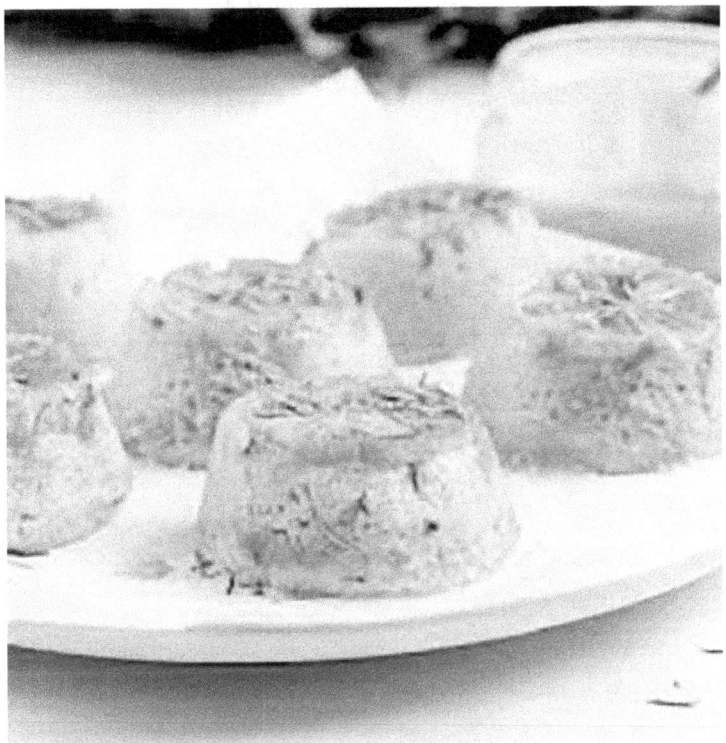

Ingredients

- » 1 teaspoon Simply Organic Pure Vanilla Extract 2 fl. oz.
- » 4 teaspoons Simply Organic Rosemary Leaf Whole 1.23 oz.
- » 1 cup butter, softened
- » 1 1/3 cups white sugar
- » 4 eggs
- » 1/2 cup sour cream

- » 4 to 5 tablespoons clementine juice (or 2 to 3 clementine's, juiced)
- » 1 tablespoon + 1 teaspoon clementine zest
- » 2 cups all-purpose flour, sifted
- » 1 teaspoon baking powder
- » 1/4 teaspoon salt
- » 8 teaspoons coconut sugar, divided
- » 16 clementine slices
- » 1/4 cup powdered sugar
- » add ingredients to cart
- » add ingredients to shopping list

Preparation

FOR THE BATTER

- » Preheat the oven to 350 degrees.
- » In a large bowl, use a mixer to beat the butter and sugar for 2 to 3 mins, until well whipped.
- » With the mixer on medium speed, add the eggs, one at a time.
- » Add the sour cream, 3 tablespoons clementine juice, 1 tablespoon clementine zest and vanilla extract. Beat for about 1 mins, until well combined, scraping the sides of the bowl if necessary.
- » Sift in the flour. Add the baking powder and salt. Stir to combine.

FOR THE TOPPING

- » On the bottom of each space in a greased cupcake or muffin pan, sprinkle 1/2 teaspoon coconut sugar and 1/4 teaspoon rosemary.

TO ASSEMBLE

- » Top the sugar and rosemary with a clementine slice, then on top of the clementine slice, using an ice cream scoop, spoon a dollop of cupcake batter.
- » Bake for 25 mins, until the cupcake batter is set. Remove the cupcakes from the muffin tin and flip upside down. The tops of the cupcakes should be slightly caramelized from the coconut sugar.
- » Allow the cupcakes to rest for 5 mins.

FOR THE ICING

- » Combine 1/4 cup powdered sugar, 1 to 2 tablespoons clementine juice and 1 teaspoon clementine zest. Mix well.
- » over tops of cupcakes, drizzle icing.
- » Serve.
- » For the icing, substitute orange juice for clementine juice, if desired.

Mango Sunrise Ice Cream with Coconut-Lime Dust

30min Duration - 20min Cook Time - 10min Prep Time

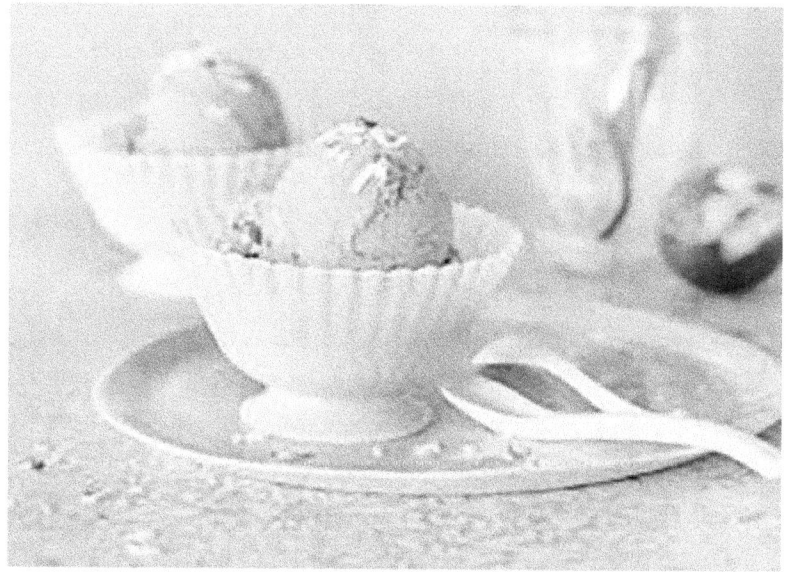

Ingredients

- 2 cups slightly thawed frozen mango chunks
- 3/4 cup coconut milk
- 1/3 cup unrefined organic cane sugar
- 1 Tbs. flaxseed oil
- 3 Tbs. dried goji berries
- ¼ cup unsweetened coconut flakes for garnish (optional)
- Zest from one lime for garnish (optional)

Preparation

- Combine mango chunks, coconut milk, cane sugar, and flax oil in a blender, and purée until very smooth. Add goji berries, and purée until finely chopped, but some visible bits remain.
- Transfer to ice cream maker, and process according to Preparation (about 20 mins). While ice cream freezes, combine coconut flakes and lime zest on cutting board, and finely chop into "dust."
- To serve, scoop ice cream into martini glasses, cups, or dessert bowls, and sprinkle with coconut-lime dust. Serve immediately.

DOMINATE

BAKLAVA CUSTARD TART

Prep Time 5m - Cook Time 10m

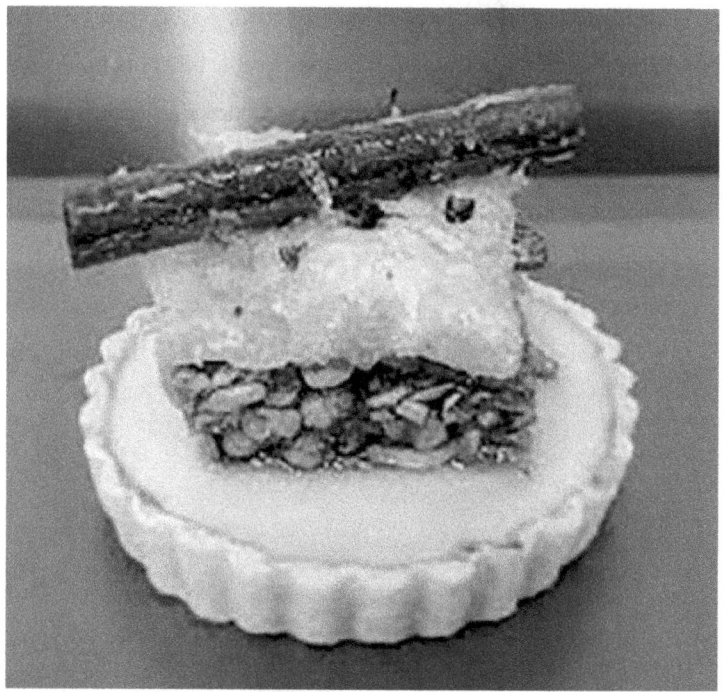

Ingredients

- » 1/2 cup firmly packed brown sugar
- » 1/3 cup light corn syrup
- » 1/4 cup Crisco® Butter Flavor All-Vegetable Shortening
- » OR 1/4 stick Crisco® Baking Sticks Butter Flavor All-Vegetable Shortening
- » 1/2 cup Jif® Creamy Peanut Butter
- » 1/4 cup milk
- » 1 teaspoon vanilla extract

Preparation

» Blend brown sugar, corn syrup and shortening in 1-quart saucepan. Cook and stir over medium-low heat until mixture just comes to a boil. Remove from heat.

» Blend in peanut butter until melted. Gradually blend in milk until mixture is smooth. Cook and stir over low heat until mixture returns to a boil. Remove from heat. Stir in vanilla. Serve warm over ice cream, cake or bread pudding.

Chocolate, Peanut Butter & Avocado Pudding

Prep: 10 Mins

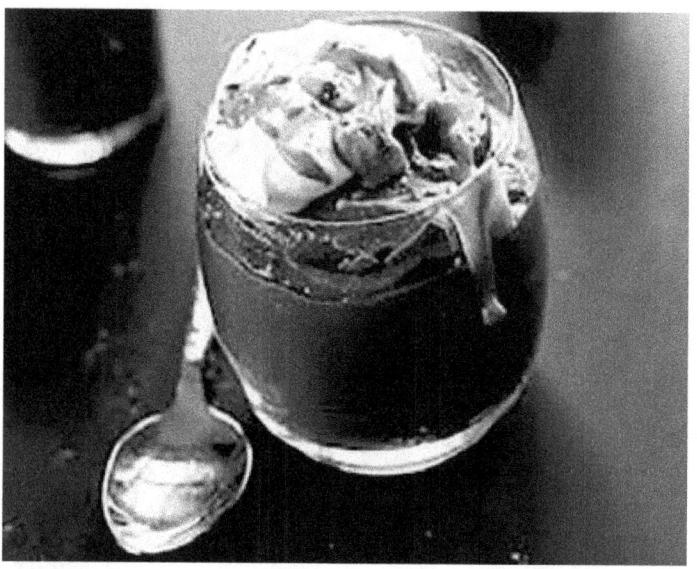

Ingredients

- 2 large, ripe avocados, halved and stoned
- 1 large banana, chopped
- 5 soft prunes
- 6 tbsp unsweetened almond milk or coconut milk
- 2 tbsp smooth peanut butter (unsweetened, if possible)
- 3 tbsp cacao powder (or good quality cocoa powder)
- 100g coconut milk yogurt (such as CoYo)
- 2 tsp maple syrup or honey
- dark chocolate
- (80% cocoa, if possible), to decorate

Preparation

- Scoop the avocado flesh into a food processor. Add the chopped banana, prunes, almond or coconut milk, smooth peanut butter and cacao powder. Blend until smooth, adding a little more milk if the blade gets stuck. Scrape down the sides once or twice and blend again.
- Divide the mixture between 4 small glasses. Mix the coconut yogurt with the maple syrup or honey and top each pudding with a generous dollop. Finely grate a little dark chocolate over the top and chill for at least 1 hr.

ORANGE & RHUBARB AMARETTI POTS

Prep: 10 Mins - Cook: 30 Mins

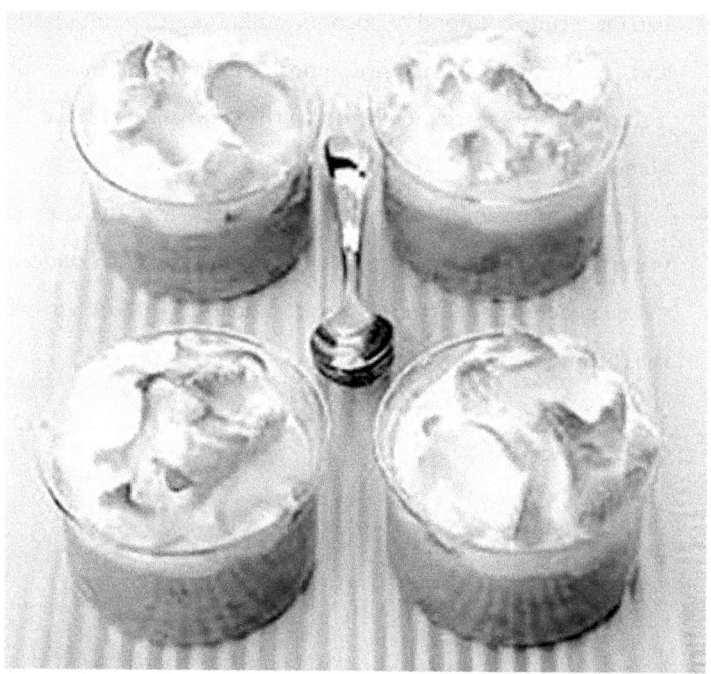

Ingredients

- » 400g double cream
- » 360g thick full-fat Greek yogurt
- » 150g amaretti biscuits, broken into small pieces
- » For the rhubarb & orange curd
- » 500g rhubarb, chopped into 2½ cm lengths
- » 150g golden caster sugar, plus a large pinch
- » 150ml orange juice, plus zest 1 orange
- » 4 medium eggs, plus 2 medium yolks
- » 150g unsalted butter

Preparation

- First, make the curd. Put the rhubarb, a pinch of sugar and the orange juice in a pan over a medium heat and cover with a lid. Cook for 10-15 mins until the rhubarb is very tender. Remove from the heat.
- Pass the rhubarb through a fine sieve, pushing it to squeeze out as much pulp as possible. Keep the flesh in the sieve to incorporate later.
- Whisk the eggs, egg yolks and sugar together until pale and frothy. Melt the butter steadily in a pan on a low heat. Once melted, slowly pour in the egg mix and orange zest, stirring continuously. Add in the strained rhubarb pulp and mix to combine, continuing to cook gently until the curd has thickened like custard. This could take 10-12 mins, but be patient and do not turn up the heat, as you might scramble the eggs.
- Once the curd has thickened, transfer it to a bowl and whisk until smooth. At this point I like to add back in the rhubarb flesh from the sieve, to give more body to the dessert – but if you want a smooth curd, don't do this.
- Whip the cream, stopping just before soft peaks start to form. Fold in the yogurt, 300g of the curd and most of the amaretti biscuits.
- Spoon the mix into eight glasses and sprinkle on the reserved amaretti. Save the remaining curd to use on pancakes, granola or to make little tartlets. Store it in a sterilized jar (wash a jar in hot soapy water, rinse, then put in the oven upside down at 120C/100C fan/gas 1/2 for 15 mins to dry).

Lemon posset with sugared-almond shortbread

Prep: 35 Mins - Cook: 30 Mins

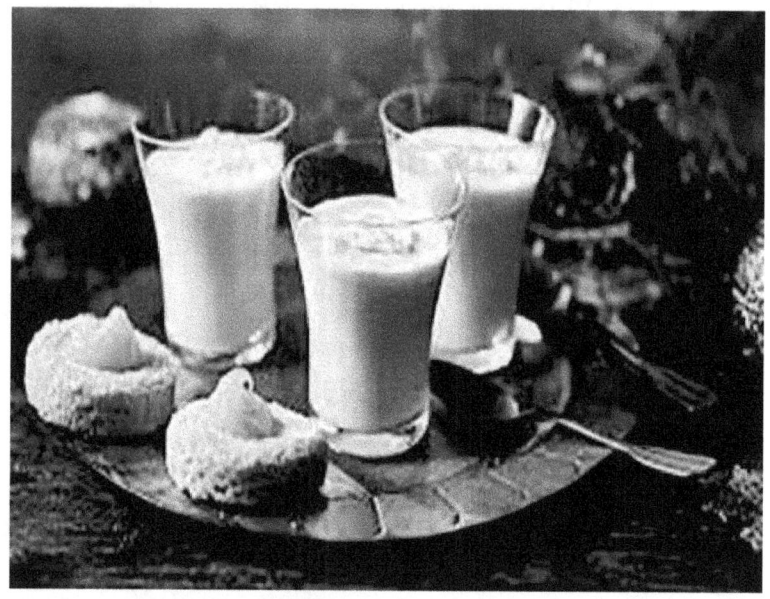

Ingredients

- 600ml double cream
- 200g golden caster sugar
- zest 3 lemons, plus 75ml juice
- For the shortbread
- 140g cold butter, diced
- 140g plain flour
- 85g golden caster sugar, plus extra for dusting
- 50g ground rice (or more flour if you can't find it)
- 85g flaked almond

Preparation

- Make the posset first. Put the cream in a big saucepan with the sugar and gently heat, stirring, until the sugar has melted. Bring to a simmer and bubble for 1 min. Turn off the heat and stir in the lemon zest and juice. Divide between pots or bowls, cool to room temperature, then carefully cover and chill for at least 3 hrs., or up to 24 hrs.
- To make the shortbread, heat oven to 160C/140C fan/gas 3. Whizz the butter and flour together in a food processor until no lumps of butter remain (or rub together with your fingertips). Tip into a bowl and stir in the sugar, ground rice and almonds. Line the base of a roughly 22cm square tin with baking parchment. Tip in the mixture and press it down firmly, making it as flat as you can. Dredge with more sugar and bake for 25-30 mins until pale golden. Cool in the tin.
- Cut the shortbread into shards and serve with the possets and little spoons.

Sauces Recipe

VEGETARIAN PASTA SAUCE

Prep: 35 Min - Cook: 2 Hours

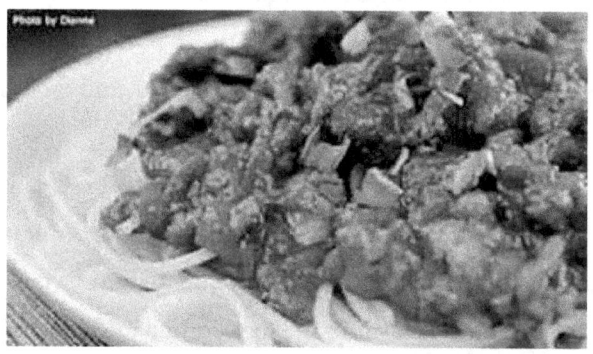

Ingredients

- 3 medium onions, chopped
- 1 medium green pepper, chopped
- 1 medium sweet red pepper, chopped
- 2 tablespoons olive oil
- 5 garlic cloves, minced
- 3 medium zucchini, chopped
- 3 medium yellow summer squash, chopped
- 3 medium tomatoes, chopped
- 1 medium eggplant, peeled and cubed
- 1/2 pound sliced fresh mushrooms
- 2 cans (28 ounces each) Italian crushed tomatoes
- 1 can (6 ounces) tomato paste
- 2 cans (2-1/4 ounces each) sliced ripe olives, drained
- 1/4 cup minced fresh basil

- » 3 tablespoons minced fresh oregano
- » 2 tablespoons minced fresh rosemary
- » 2 teaspoons Italian seasoning
- » 1-1/2 teaspoons salt
- » 1/2 teaspoon pepper

Preparation

- » In a Dutch oven, saute the onions and peppers in oil until tender. Add garlic; cook 1 mins longer. Add the zucchini, summer squash, tomatoes, eggplant and mushrooms; cook and stir for 5 mins.
- » Stir in the remaining ingredients. Bring to a boil. Reduce heat; simmer, uncovered, for 1-1/2 to 2 hours or until sauce is thickened.

Mumbo Sauce

Total: 25 Mins - Prep: 10 Mins - Cook: 15 Mins

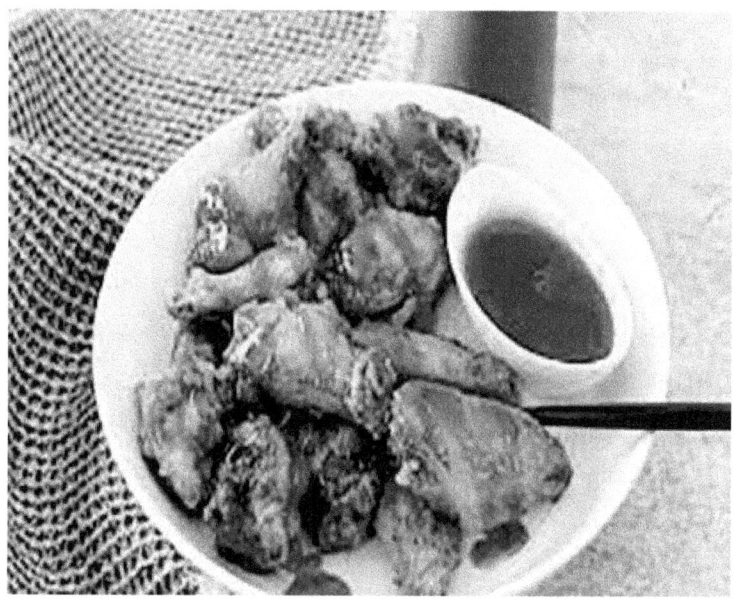

Ingredients

- 1 cup ketchup
- 3/4 cup cane syrup (such as Steen's or Lyle's Golden Syrup)
- 1/4 cup granulated sugar
- 1/3 cup white vinegar
- 1/4 cup water
- 2 tablespoons soy sauce
- 1/2 teaspoon sweet, mild paprika
- 1/2 teaspoon hot sauce (or more for a hot version)
- Dash kosher salt

Preparation

- Gather the ingredients.
- ingredients for mumbo sauce
- Combine all of the ingredients in a saucepan and whisk to blend.
- mumbo sweet and sour sauce in a saucepan
- Bring the sauce mixture to a simmer over medium heat. Turn the heat down to low and continue to cook, occasionally stirring, for about 15 mins.
- umbo sauce simmering
- Let the sauce cool and then pour it into a container or squeeze bottle; label with the name and date. Keep the sauce refrigerated and use within 2 weeks.
- jar of mumbo sauce
- Serve the sauce with chicken wings, egg rolls, or use it as a glaze or barbecue sauce for meatloaf, ribs, chops, or chicken.

TACO SAUCE

Total: 17 Mins - Prep: 2 Mins - Cook: 15 Mins

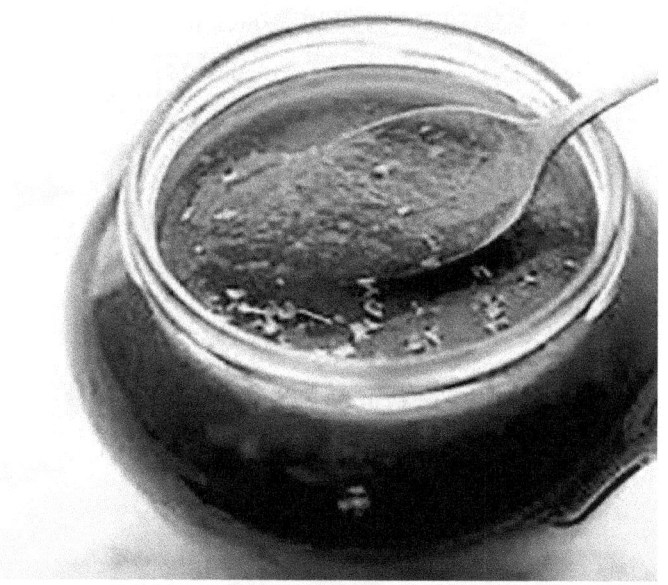

Ingredients

- 1 (16-ounce) can tomato sauce
- 1 (8-ounce) can diced tomatoes and green chiles
- 1 (4-ounce) can diced jalapenos
- 2 tablespoons vinegar (white or apple cider)
- 1 tablespoon ground cumin
- 1 teaspoon ground coriander
- 1 tablespoon garlic (minced)
- 1 teaspoon salt

- » 1 teaspoon chili powder
- » 1/4 teaspoon cayenne powder
- » 1 teaspoon paprika
- » 1 teaspoon white sugar
- » 1/2 cup water

Preparation

- » Add all of the ingredients to a high-speed blender.
- » Blend until completely smooth. Add more water if the sauce is too thick.
- » Add the sauce to a saucepan and heat on medium for 10 to 15 mins. Stir frequently to avoid any burning on the bottom of the pan. Add more salt to taste.
- » Allow the sauce to cool, then place it in a glass bottle or jar and store it in the refrigerator. You can also bottle or can it using a canning technique.
- » Serve it up on tacos, nachos, or anything that needs taco sauce!

Creamy Jalapeno Sauce

Prep: 15 Mins - Cook: 15 Mins

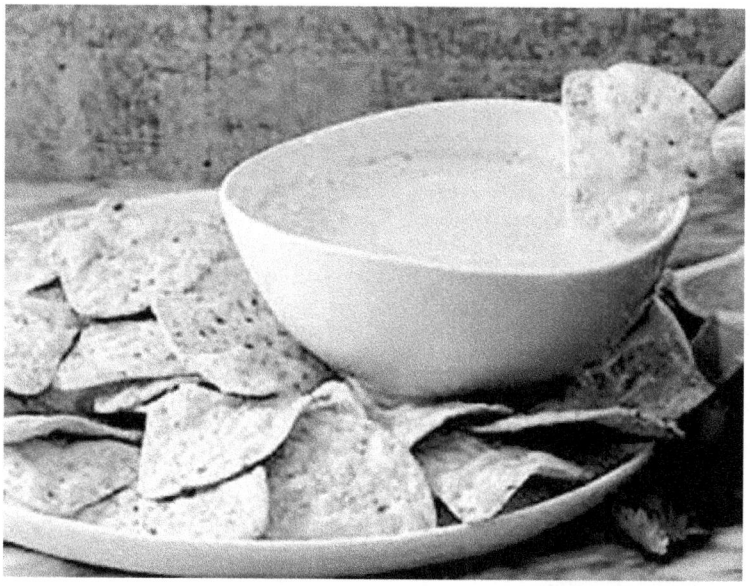

Ingredients

- 1 cup sour cream
- 1 cup mayonnaise
- 1/3 cup buttermilk
- 1/2 cup cilantro (packed)
- 1/2 cup pickled jalapeño pepper rings, plus 3 tablespoons of the juice
- 1 (1-ounce) packet dry ranch dressing mix
- 1/2 teaspoon garlic powder
- Pinch kosher salt (or to taste)
- 1 tablespoon lime juice
- Optional: 2 tablespoons tomatillo salsa

Preparation

- In a bowl, combine the sour cream, mayonnaise, buttermilk, cilantro, jalapeño pepper rings and juice, ranch dressing mix, garlic powder, a pinch of salt, and the lime juice. Stir to blend.
- Creamy jalapeno sauce ingredients in a bowl
- Pour the sauce mixture into a blender or food processor and pulse until smooth. Taste and add the tomatillo salsa, if using, or add extra jalapeño pickle juice or buttermilk to thin.
- Creamy jalapeno sauce in a blender
- Pour the dip into a container or jars and refrigerate until serving time.
- Jalapeno sauce in jars
- Serve creamy jalapeño sauce in a small bowl with poppers, chicken wings, tortilla chips, or quesadillas.
- Creamy jalapeno dip with poppers and mozzarella sticks

Roasted Tomato Sauce

Total: 95 Mins - Prep: 20 Mins - Cook: 75 Mins

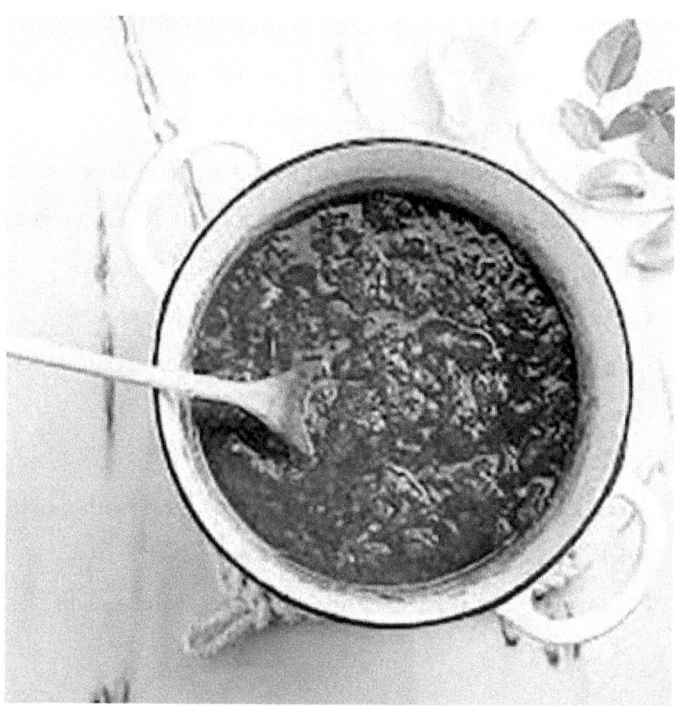

Ingredients

- 3 pounds tomatoes
- 3 tablespoons extra-virgin olive oil
- 6 cloves garlic (peeled, sliced)
- 1/2 cup onion or shallot (sliced)
- 2 teaspoons Italian seasoning
- 1 teaspoon kosher salt (or to taste)
- 1/4 teaspoon black pepper (freshly ground)
- 2 to 3 tablespoons basil (chopped)
- Optional: 2 to 3 tablespoons tomato paste

- » Optional: 1/8 teaspoon crushed red pepper flakes
- » Optional: 1 pound pasta (e.g., bucatini, spaghetti, linguine)

Preparation

- » preheat the oven to 325 F.
- » Cut the cores out of large tomatoes; slice or chop the tomatoes into 1-inch to 2-inch chunks.
- » Chop the tomatoes.
- » Toss the tomatoes in a large bowl with the olive oil, sliced garlic, onion, Italian seasoning, salt, and black pepper.
- » Tomatoes cut up in a bowl.
- » Arrange the tomatoes in a single layer on a large rimmed baking sheet. Roast the tomatoes for 1 hour.
- » Put the roasted tomatoes and seasonings through a food mill; this will eliminate the skins and most of the seeds to make a smooth sauce. If you don't have a food mill, process the mixture in a blender or food processor.
- » Put the roasted tomatoes through a food mill.
- » Transfer the tomato mixture to a large saucepan and add the basil. Add the tomato paste and red pepper flakes, if using. Bring the sauce to a simmer; reduce the heat to low and simmer for about 15 mins, or until slightly reduced and thickened.
- » Simmer the tomato sauce with the fresh basil.
- » Cook the pasta in boiling salted water, if using; drain, but do not rinse. Toss the hot drained pasta with the sauce. Serve with garlic bread, if desired.
- » Bucatini with roasted tomato sauce.
- » If not using immediately, pour the sauce into containers or jars with lids. Refrigerate the sauce and use within 3 days or store it in the freezer for up to 4 months.

Tomato Sauce with Fresh Vegetables and Basil

110 Mins - Prep:20 Mins - Cook:90 Mins

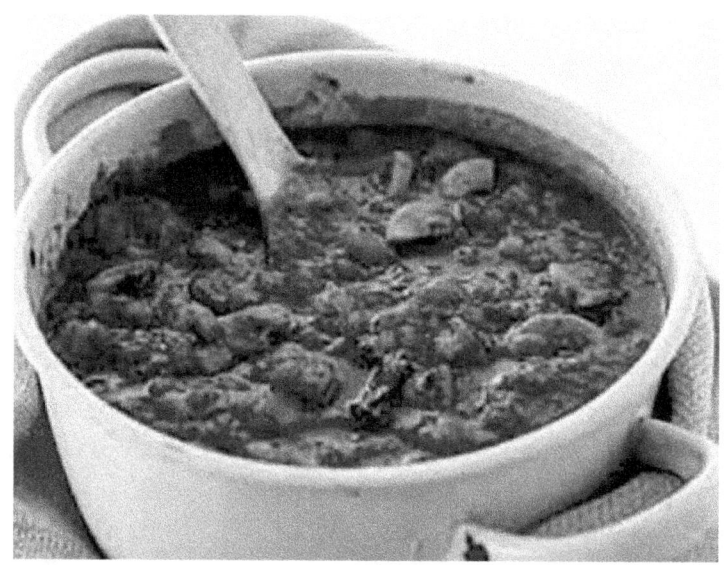

Ingredients

- 3/4 cup chopped onion
- 2 cloves garlic (crushed and minced)
- 3 tablespoons olive oil
- 6 cups chopped tomatoes (canned or about 6 fresh peeled tomatoes)
- 3/4 cup dry red wine
- 1/4 cup shredded carrots
- 1/4 cup chopped parsley (fresh)
- 1/3 cup chopped basil (fresh)
- 1 teaspoon granulated sugar

- 1 teaspoon salt
- 1 cup zucchini (sliced)
- 1 cup mushrooms (sliced)

Preparation

- Heat olive oil in Dutch oven over medium heat; add onion, cooking until tender. Stir in garlic, tomatoes, wine, carrots, parsley, basil, sugar, and salt.
- Bring sauce to a boil. Reduce heat and simmer, uncovered, for 1 hour, stirring frequently.
- Add sliced zucchini and mushrooms; cook until sauce is thick, about 20 mins longer. Serve with hot cooked pasta.

Sweet Potato Dip

Total: 55 Mins - Prep: 10 Mins - Cook: 45 Mins

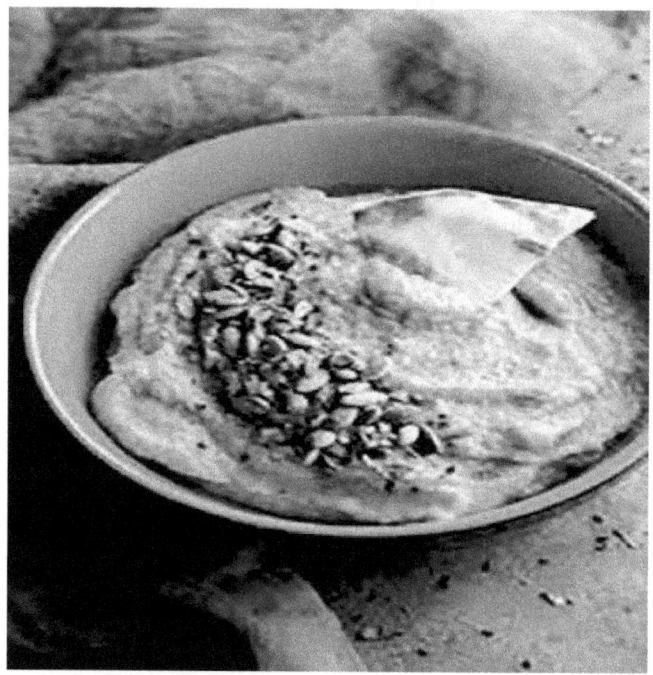

Ingredients

- » 1 large sweet potato
- » 1 clove garlic
- » 1/4 cup raw almond butter (or seed or nut butter of your choice)
- » 1/2 teaspoon smoked paprika
- » 1/4 to 1/2 teaspoon cayenne pepper
- » Dash sea salt (to taste)
- » Fresh lemon juice to taste

Preparation

- Gather the ingredients.
- Preheat an oven to 425 F.
- Scrub the sweet potato clean and put it in the oven to roast until it's tender when pierced with a fork, about 45 mins. Alternatively, you can cook the sweet potato in a microwave—poke the sweet potato all over with a fork and microwave on high in 1-mins increments until the sweet potato is tender all the way through, about 6 mins total.
- When the sweet potato is done, let it sit at room temperature until it's cool enough to handle, at least 30 mins. Remove and discard the peel and put the roasted, peeled sweet potato in a food processor. Pulse a few times just to start to break the sweet potato down.
- Peel and mince the garlic and add it to the sweet potato. Pulse to combine. Add in the almond butter, smoked paprika, and cayenne pepper, to the sweet potato. Whirl, scraping the sides of the bowl down with a spatula as necessary to keep the mixture together until the mixture is silky smooth.
- Add salt and lemon juice to taste. Transfer the mixture to a serving bowl. Serve immediately or cover and chill for up to 3 days.

Vegetarian Crock Pot Spaghetti Sauce

Total: 8hrs. 35 mins - prep:35 mins - cook:8 hrs.

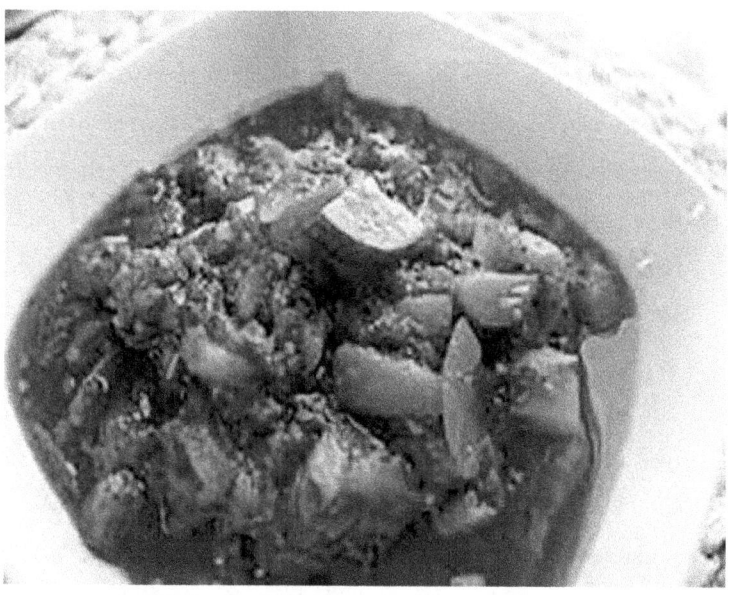

Ingredients

- 2 tbsp. olive oil
- 1 onion (chopped)
- 3 cloves garlic (minced)
- 2 carrots (one chopped, one shredded)
- 1 (8-ounce) package sliced mushrooms
- 1 green bell pepper (chopped)
- 15 oz. can tomato sauce
- 2 (14 oz.) cans of diced tomatoes (undrained)
- 6 oz. can tomato paste
- 1 tsp. dried Italian seasoning

- » 1/4 tsp. pepper
- » 1/2 tsp. salt
- » 2 tsp. sugar
- » 16 oz. box spaghetti

Preparation

- » Gather the ingredients.
- » Add the olive oil to a large skillet and heat over medium heat.
- » Add the onions and garlic and cook, stirring frequently, for 4 to 5 mins until they are tender.
- » Add the carrots, mushrooms, and bell pepper and stir.
- » Cook for another 2 to 3 mins.
- » Place the vegetables in the bottom of a 4 to 5-quart crock pot and add the tomato sauce, diced tomatoes, tomato paste, Italian seasoning, pepper, salt, and sugar.
- » Stir well.
- » Cover the crock pot and cook on low for 7 to 8 hours. This recipe can cook as long as 10 hours.
- » Uncover the slow cooker, stir the sauce thoroughly, then leave the cover off the crockpot and turn the heat to high.
- » Cook, uncovered, for 1 to 2 more hours to thicken the sauce.
- » At this point, the sauce can be frozen.
- » Or you can go ahead and serve the heated sauce with cooked spaghetti and grated parmesan cheese.

Easy Cherry Sauce

Total:10 Mins - Prep:5 Mins - Cook:5 Mins

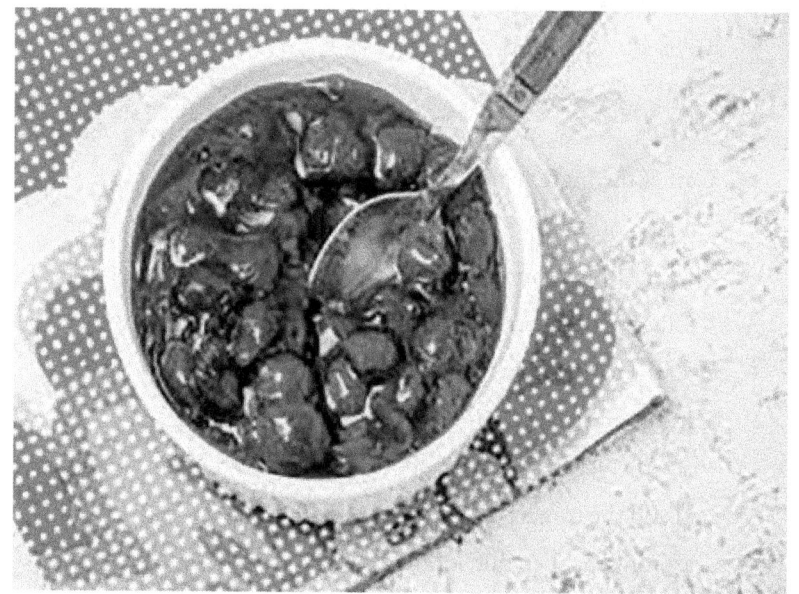

Ingredients

- » 16 ounces cherries (frozen or fresh, pitted)
- » 1/2 cup granulated sugar
- » 1/2 cup water
- » 1 tablespoon cornstarch
- » 1 tablespoon lemon juice (fresh)

Preparation

- Gather the ingredients.
- Cherry Sauce Ingredients (cherries, lemon, sugar, water, corn starch)
- In a medium saucepan, bring the cherries, sugar, and water to a boil over medium-high heat, stirring often.
- Cherry mix boiling in a pot
- In a small bowl, stir the lemon juice and cornstarch together until smooth.
- Cornstarch and lemon juice in a cup
- Whisk it into the boiling cherry mixture.
- Return to a boil, stirring constantly. You don't want this sauce to scorch on the bottom.
- Stirring cherry sauce in a pot
- Cook until the liquid has thickened, which should take about 1 more mins.
- Remove the pot from the heat and taste. You can add a little extra sugar or lemon juice if needed at this point, depending on your personal preference.
- Allow the sauce to cool to room temperature and serve over ice cream or cheesecake.

Chapter 10

SNACKS AND SMOOTHIES RECIPES

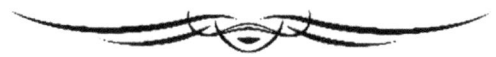

TOMATO DIP WITH GRILLED BREAD

Prep Time: 10 Mins - Cook Time: 5 Mins

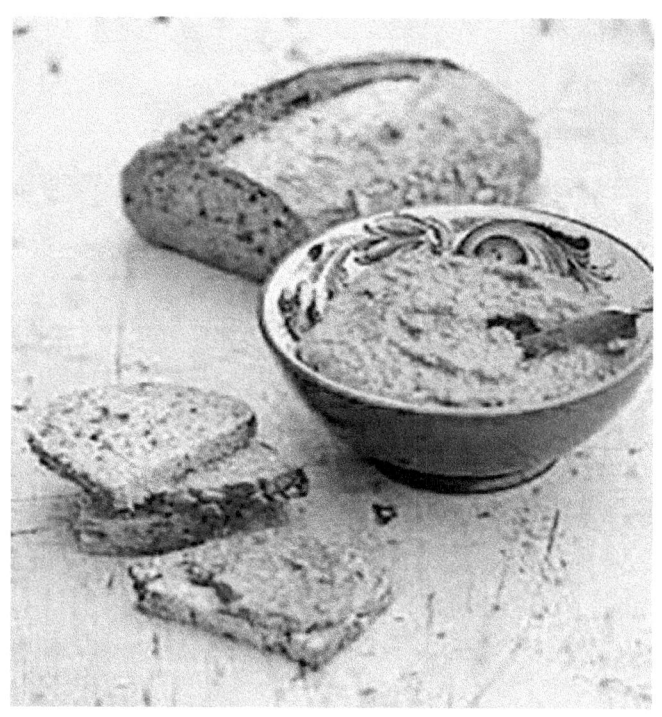

Ingredients

- For the famous tomato dip
- 3/4 cup roasted almonds
- 15-ounce can crush fire roasted tomatoes
- 1 garlic clove
- 1/2 teaspoon kosher salt
- 1/4 cup olive oil
- For the grilled bread
- 1 baguette or artisan loaf (like our artisan Dutch oven bread)
- Olive oil

Preparation

- In the bowl of a food processor, combine the roasted almonds, fire roasted tomatoes, garlic, and kosher salt. Process until the nuts are finely ground.
- Scrape down the bowl. With the processor running, add the olive oil in a steady stream until a thick texture forms. (Store any leftovers refrigerated for 1 week.)
- For the grilled bread: Slice the baguette into slices. Brush olive oil onto each side of the bread. In a grill pan or on a grill, toast each bread slice over medium high heat until browned, a few mins per side.

Sweet & Spicy Roasted Party Nuts

Prep Time: 10 Mins - Cook Time: 25 Mins - Total Time: 35 Mins

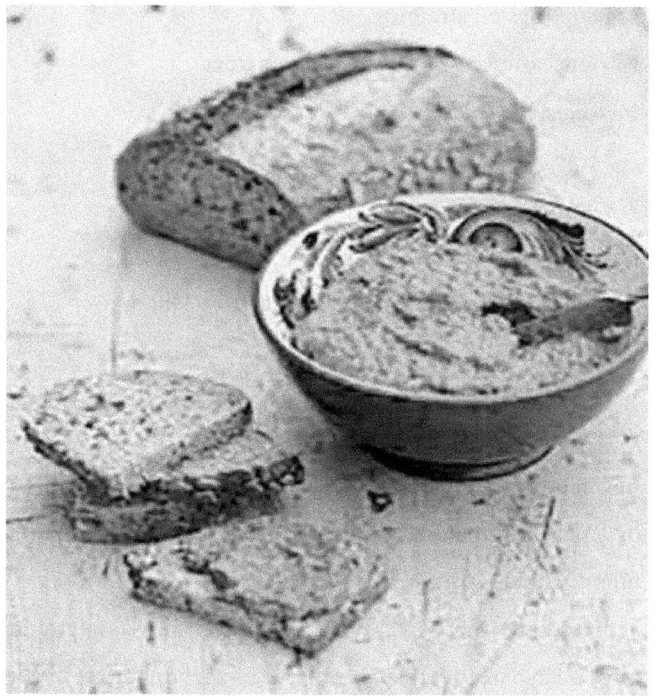

Ingredients

- » 2 cups whole almonds
- » 2 cups pecan or walnut halves
- » 1 ½ cup pepitas (green pumpkin seeds)
- » Optional but so good: 2 tablespoons finely snipped or chopped fresh rosemary (from 4 big sprigs)
- » 2 tablespoons maple syrup
- » 2 tablespoons unsalted butter, melted
- » 1 ½ teaspoons kosher salt*

- » 1 teaspoon vanilla extract
- » ¼ teaspoon cayenne pepper (reduce or omit if sensitive to spice)

Preparation

- » Preheat the oven to 325 degrees Fahrenheit. Line a large rimmed baking sheet with parchment paper or a silicone baking mat so the maple syrup doesn't get stuck to the pan (this is important). Pour the almonds, pecans and pepitas onto the pan and set it aside.
- » In a small bowl, combine the optional rosemary (or any other added seasonings), maple syrup, melted butter, salt, vanilla, and cayenne (if you using). Gently whisk until blended.
- » Pour the mixture over the nuts on the prepared baking sheet. Stir well, until all of the nuts are lightly coated. Spread the mixture in a single layer across the pan (the maple syrup will pool on the bottom of the pan, but that's okay).
- » Bake, stirring after the first 10 mins and then every 5 mins thereafter, until almost no maple syrup remains on the parchment paper and the nuts are deeply golden, 23 to 26 mins. (The maple syrup coating will be a little sticky right out of the oven, but will harden as the pecans cool.)
- » Remove the pan from the oven and stir the nuts one more time, spreading them into an even layer across the pan. Let them cool down for about 10 mins, then, while the nuts are still warm, carefully separate any large clumps (this may or may not be necessary).

» Let the nut mixture cool completely on the pan. These will keep for up to 2 months in a sealed bag at room temperature.

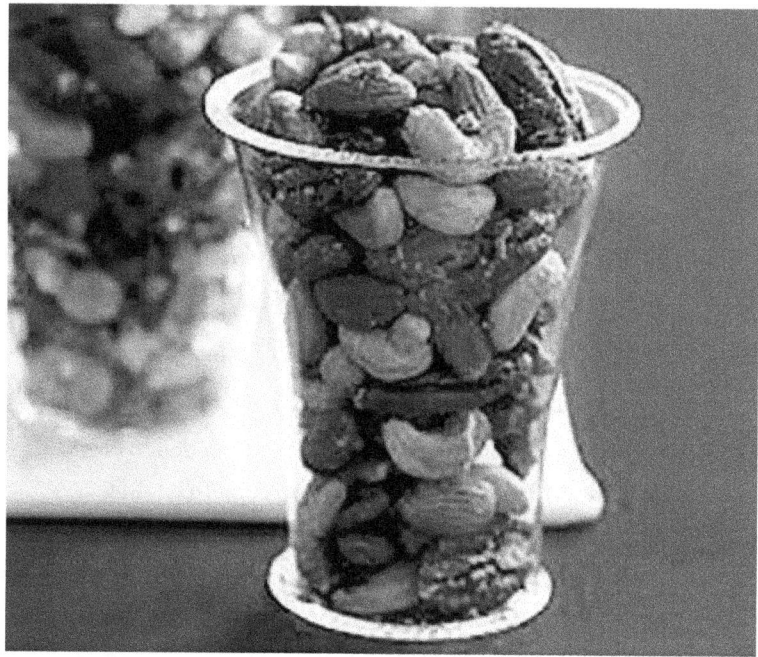

Roasted Cauliflower

Prep Time: 10 mins - Cook Time: 30 mins - Total Time: 40 mins

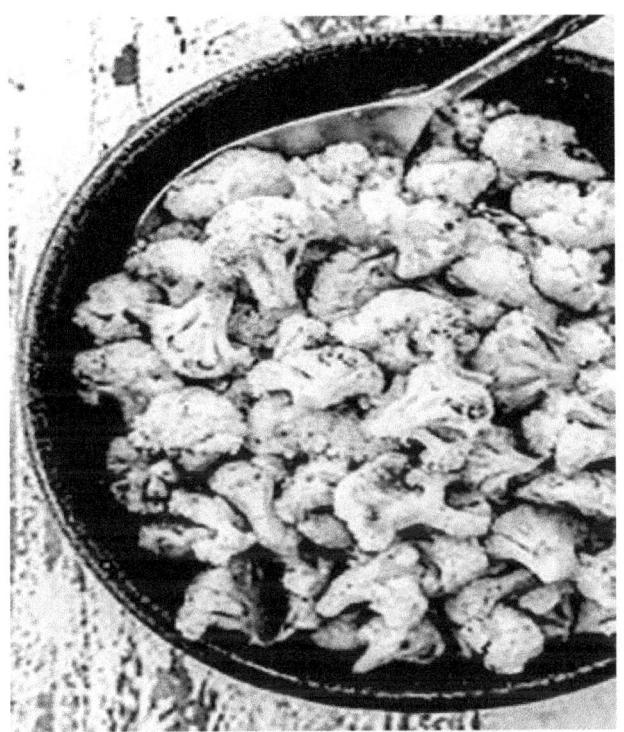

Ingredients

- Basic roasted cauliflower
- 1 large head of cauliflower
- 2 to 3 tablespoons extra-virgin olive oil, as needed
- ¼ teaspoon fine sea salt
- Freshly ground black pepper, to taste

Perfect Roasted Sweet Potatoes

Prep Time: 10 Mins - Cook Time: 30 Mins - Total Time: 40 Mins

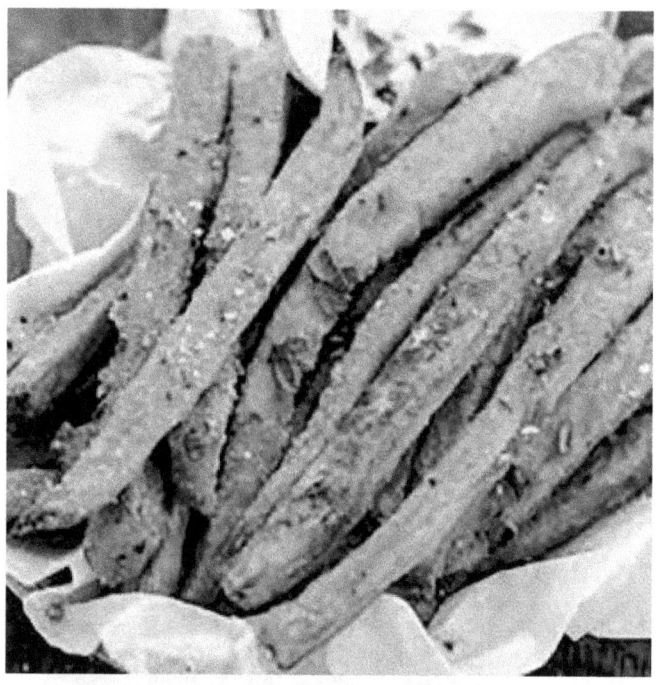

Ingredients

- » 2 pounds sweet potatoes (3 to 4 medium sweet potatoes)
- » 2 tablespoons extra-virgin olive oil
- » Optional: 1 teaspoon chili powder or freshly ground black pepper, to taste
- » ¼ teaspoon fine sea salt

Preparation

- Preheat the oven to 425 degrees Fahrenheit and line a large, rimmed baking sheet with parchment paper for easy clean-up.
- Either scrub the sweet potatoes clean and pat dry, or peel them (I generally peel mine). To slice, use a sharp chef's knife to cut them into 1-inch thick rounds. Then, cut up each round to make 1-inch cubes. The "cubes" won't be perfectly even, but that's ok.
- Place the sweet potatoes on the prepared baking sheet. Drizzle the olive oil on top. If using, sprinkle the chili pepper or several twists of freshly ground black pepper on top, followed by the salt. Toss until the sweet potatoes are all evenly coated in oil, and arrange them in a single layer.
- Bake for 30 to 40 mins, tossing halfway, until the sweet potatoes are tender and caramelizing at the edges. Serve while warm. Leftover sweet potatoes will keep in the refrigerator, covered, for about 4 days. Gently reheat in the microwave or oven if desired.

Easy Pineapple Mint Popsicles

Prep Time: 5 Mins - Total Time: 5 Mins

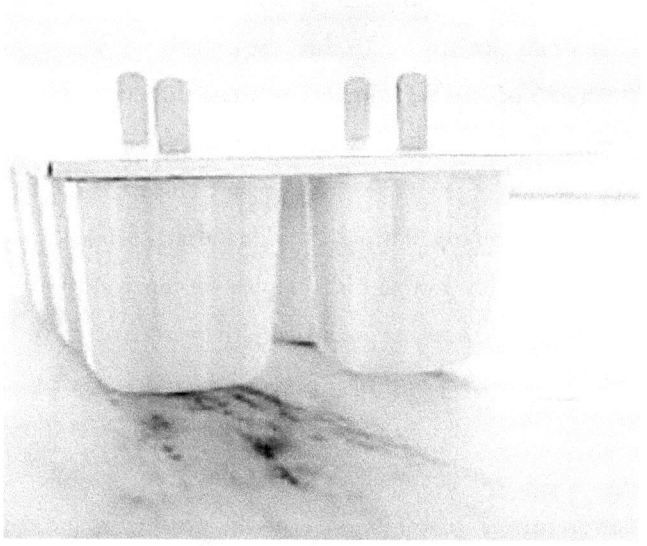

Ingredients

- » 1 pound frozen pineapple chunks, defrosted completely in the refrigerator
- » 1 tablespoon lightly packed fresh mint leaves, to taste

Preparation

- » In a blender, combine the thawed pineapple and mint. Blend until completely smooth. Taste, and add a few more mint leaves if you'd prefer more minty flavor. Blend again.
- » Pour the mixture into your popsicle molds, insert popsicle sticks. Freeze until frozen solid. Enjoy!

Sweet & Spicy Roasted Party Nuts

Prep Time: 10 Mins - Cook Time: 25 Mins - Total Time: 35 Mins

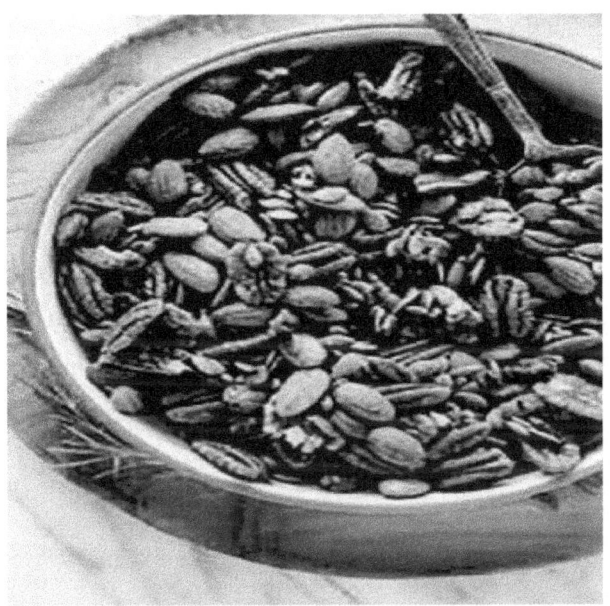

Ingredients

- 2 cups whole almonds
- 2 cups pecan or walnut halves
- 1 ½ cup pepitas (green pumpkin seeds)
- Optional but so good: 2 tablespoons finely snipped or chopped fresh rosemary (from 4 big sprigs)
- 2 tablespoons maple syrup
- 2 tablespoons unsalted butter, melted
- 1 ½ teaspoons kosher salt*
- 1 teaspoon vanilla extract
- ¼ teaspoon cayenne pepper (reduce or omit if sensitive to spice)

Preparation

- Preheat the oven to 325 degrees Fahrenheit. Line a large rimmed baking sheet with parchment paper or a silicone baking mat so the maple syrup doesn't get stuck to the pan (this is important). Pour the almonds, pecans and pepitas onto the pan and set it aside.
- In a small bowl, combine the optional rosemary (or any other added seasonings), maple syrup, melted butter, salt, vanilla, and cayenne (if you using). Gently whisk until blended.
- Pour the mixture over the nuts on the prepared baking sheet. Stir well, until all of the nuts are lightly coated. Spread the mixture in a single layer across the pan (the maple syrup will pool on the bottom of the pan, but that's okay).
- Bake, stirring after the first 10 mins and then every 5 mins thereafter, until almost no maple syrup remains on the parchment paper and the nuts are deeply golden, 23 to 26 mins. (The maple syrup coating will be a little sticky right out of the oven, but will harden as the pecans cool.)
- Remove the pan from the oven and stir the nuts one more time, spreading them into an even layer across the pan. Let them cool down for about 10 mins, then, while the nuts are still warm, carefully separate any large clumps (this may or may not be necessary).
- Let the nut mixture cool completely on the pan. These will keep for up to 2 months in a sealed bag at room temperature.

The Best Guacamole

Prep Time: 15 Mins - Total Time: 15 Mins

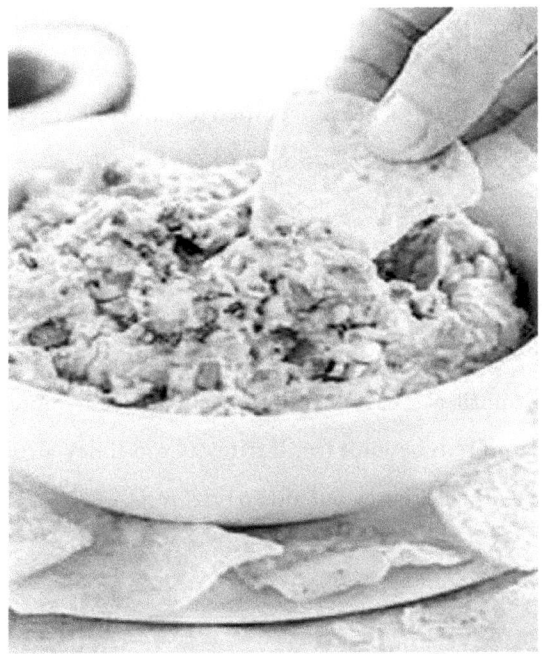

Ingredients

- 4 medium ripe avocados, halved and pitted
- ½ cup finely chopped white onion (about ½ small onion)
- ¼ cup finely chopped fresh cilantro
- 1 small jalapeño, seeds and ribs removed, finely chopped
- 3 tablespoons lime juice (from about 1 ½ limes), or more if needed
- ¼ teaspoon ground coriander
- 1 teaspoon kosher salt, more to taste

PREPARATION

» Using a spoon, scoop the flesh of the avocados into a low serving bowl, discarding any bruised, browned areas.

» Using a pastry cutter, potato masher, or fork, mash up the avocado until it reaches your desired texture (I like my guacamole to have some texture, so I stop mashing once there are just small chunks remaining).

» Promptly add the onion, cilantro, jalapeño, lime juice, coriander, and salt. Stir to combine.

» Taste and add additional salt (I often add up to ½ teaspoon more), until the flavors really sing. If it needs more zip, add a little more lime juice (or, if it tastes too limey already, don't worry—it will mellow out after a brief rest).

Perfect Roasted Broccoli

Prep Time: 5 Mins - Cook Time: 20 Mins - Total Time: 25 Mins

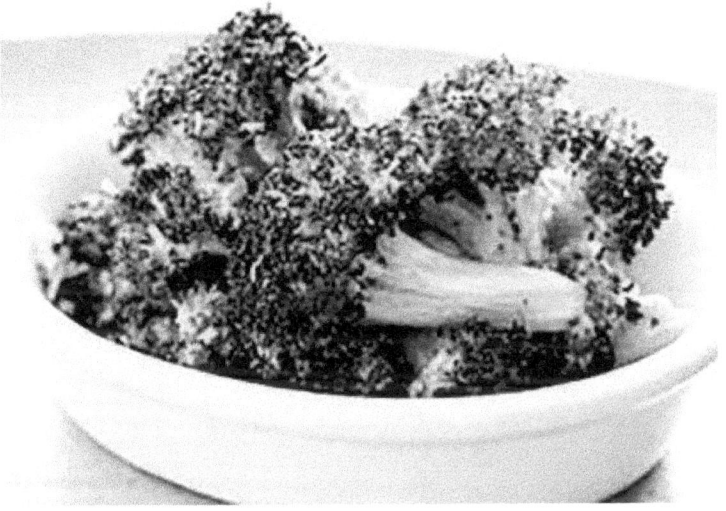

Ingredients

- 1 pound (16 ounces) broccoli florets, cut into bite-sized pieces (from 2 pounds or about 1 ½ bunches of broccoli)
- 2 tablespoons extra-virgin olive oil
- Salt and freshly ground black pepper

Preparation

- Preheat the oven to 425 degrees Fahrenheit. Line a large, rimmed baking sheet for easy clean-up, if desired.
- On the prepared baking sheet, toss the broccoli with the oil until all of the florets are lightly coated. Arrange them in an even layer across the pan, then sprinkle salt and pepper on top.

» Bake for 18 to 22 mins, tossing halfway, or until the florets are turning deeply golden on the edges. Season to taste with additional salt and pepper, if necessary, and serve warm.

Garlic Herb White Bean Dip

Prep Time: 10 Mins

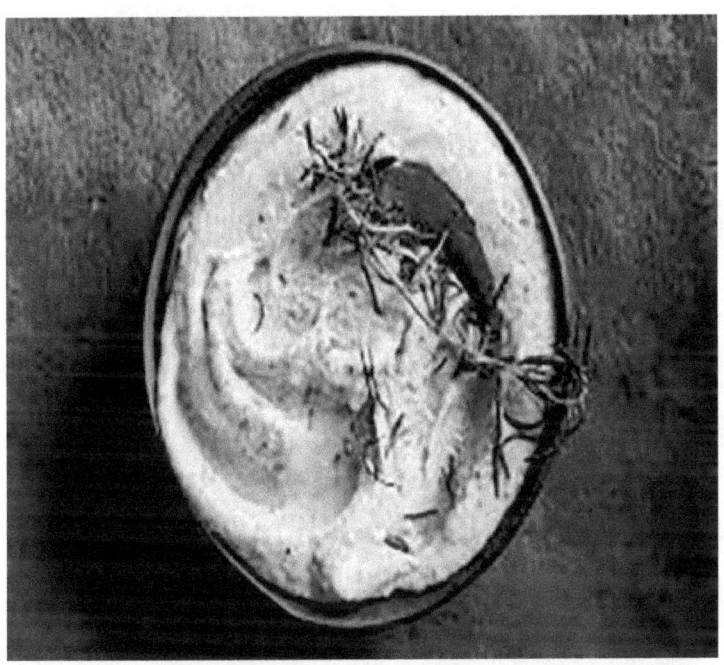

Ingredients

- 1 medium garlic clove
- 1/2 cup packed fresh herbs (basil, thyme, oregano, chives, a small amount of rosemary leaves)
- 2 15-ounce cans cannellini beans
- 1/2 cup olive oil
- 2 tablespoons white wine vinegar
- 3/4 teaspoon kosher salt
- Freshly ground black pepper

- » To serve: carrots, celery, veggies, crackers, bread, pita, pita chips, homemade crackers, or crostini

Preparation

- » Peel the garlic. Remove any tough stems from the herbs; measure out 1/2 cup (remember with rosemary, a little goes a long way). Drain and rinse the white beans.
- » In the bowl of a food processor, add garlic and herbs and process until finely chopped.
  Add the white beans, olive oil, white wine vinegar, kosher salt, and black pepper. Process until smooth, scraping down the bowl as necessary. Store in the refrigerator for up to 1 week.

Aji Verde (Spicy Peruvian Green Sauce)

Prep Time: 10 Mins - Total Time: 10 Mins

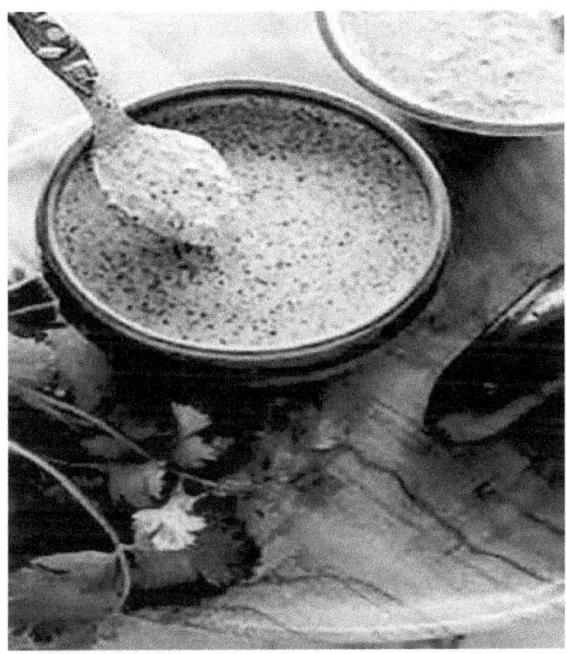

Ingredients

- ½ cup mayonnaise (I love Sir Kensington's brand)
- 2 cups lightly packed fresh cilantro, mostly leaves but small stems are ok (from 1 big bunch of cilantro or 1 ½ medium)
- 2 medium jalapeños, seeds and membranes removed but reserved, roughly chopped
- 2 cloves garlic, roughly chopped
- ⅓ cup (1 ounce) grated Cotija or Parmesan cheese
- 1 tablespoon lime juice
- ¼ teaspoon fine sea salt

Preparation

- In a food processor or blender, combine all of the ingredients. Blend until the cilantro has broken into very tiny pieces and the sauce is green and mostly smooth (no matter how long you blend it, it will still have some texture to it).
- Taste, and adjust if necessary. This sauce is intentionally bold and spicy and I usually think it's just right as written. However, if the flavor is too overwhelming, blend in 1 tablespoon of olive oil while running the food processor. If it's not spicy enough, add some of the reserved jalapeño seeds and blend again. If it doesn't have enough zip, add another tablespoon of lime juice and/or a pinch of salt.

Honey Butter Cornbread

Prep Time: 10 Mins - Cook Time: 35 Mins - Total Time: 45 Mins

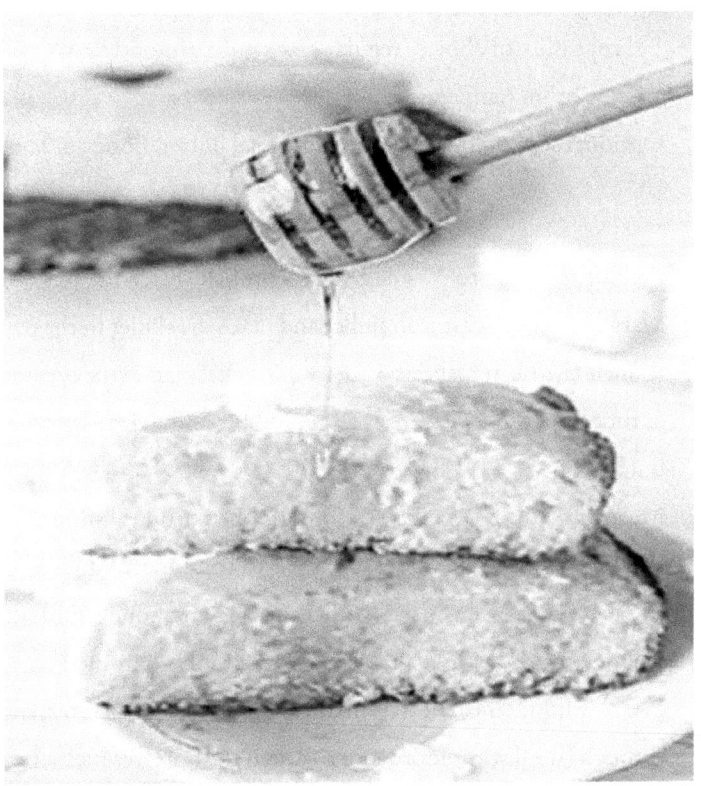

Ingredients

- ½ cup (1 stick) unsalted butter
- 1 ½ cups cornmeal, medium-grind or finer*
- 1 ½ cups white whole wheat flour, regular whole wheat flour or all-purpose flour
- 1 ½ teaspoons fine sea salt
- 2 teaspoons baking powder

- » ½ teaspoon baking soda
- » 3 large eggs, at room temperature**
- » ⅔ cup honey or maple syrup
- » 1 ½ cups milk of choice (regular cow's milk, almond or oat milk, etc.), at room temperature
- » Optional serving suggestions: additional butter, honey or jam

Preparation

- » Preheat the oven to 375 degrees Fahrenheit. Place the butter in a large (12-inch) cast iron skillet and place the skillet in the oven to melt the butter, about 5 to 13 mins (keep an extra eye on it as time goes on—we want it to get bubbly and lightly browned, but not burnt).
- » Meanwhile, in a large bowl, combine the cornmeal, flour, salt, baking powder and baking soda. Stir to combine, and set aside. In a medium bowl, whisk together the eggs and honey until fully blended. Add the milk and whisk until evenly combined.
- » Pour the liquid into the dry mixture, and stir just until moistened through (we'll stir it more soon). When the butter is melted and golden, use oven mitts (the skillet is crazy hot!) to remove the skillet from the oven, and give it a gentle swirl to lightly coat about an inch up the sides.
- » Pour the melted butter into the batter and stir just until incorporated. Return the skillet to the oven and bake until the bread is brown around the edge, springy to the touch, and a toothpick inserted in the center comes out clean with just a few crumbs, 25 to 30 mins. Carefully (with oven mitts), place the

skillet on a cooling rack. Let it cool for at least 5 mins before slicing and serving—perhaps with extra butter, honey or jam on the side.

» This cornbread will keep at room temperature in a sealed container for up to 3 days, or up to a week in the refrigerator. You can also freeze it for up to 3 months. Gently reheat before serving.

Easy Pineapple Mint Popsicles

Prep Time: 5 Mins - Total Time: 5 Mins (Plus Thawing/Freezing Time)

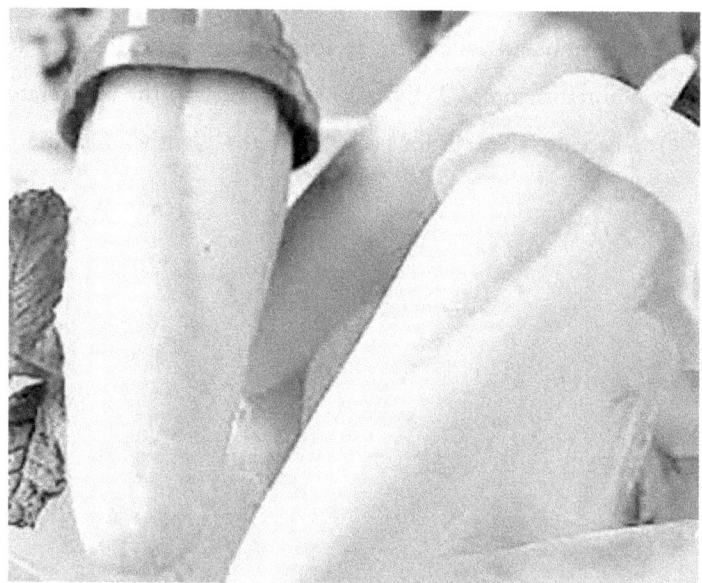

Ingredients

- » 1-pound frozen pineapple chunks, defrosted completely in the refrigerator
- » 1 tablespoon lightly packed fresh mint leaves, to taste

Preparation

- » In a blender, combine the thawed pineapple and mint. Blend until completely smooth. Taste, and add a few more mint leaves if you'd prefer more minty flavor. Blend again.
- » Pour the mixture into your popsicle molds, insert popsicle sticks. Freeze until frozen solid. Enjoy

Easy Green Goddess Dressing

Prep Time: 5 Mins - Total Time: 5 Mins

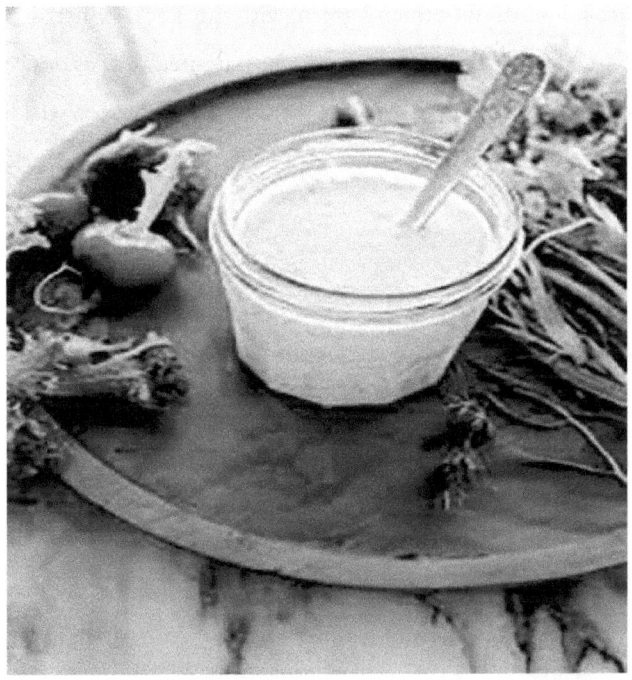

Ingredients

- » 1 cup plain Greek yogurt, preferably full-fat (made with whole milk)
- » 1 cup lightly packed fresh herbs (tender stems are fine): use cilantro, parsley, dill, basil and/or mint, with up to ¼ cup chives or green onion (sliced into ½" segments)
- » Optional: Up to 2 tablespoons fresh tarragon leaves
- » 1 medium clove garlic, roughly chopped
- » ½ teaspoon fine sea salt
- » Lots of freshly ground black pepper, to taste

Preparation

- Combine all of the ingredients in the bowl of a food processor. Process until smooth and green, with tiny flecks of herbs.
- Taste, and add more salt or pepper if desired. Use as desired, or cover and refrigerate for later. This dressing will keep well in the fridge for 5 to 7 days.

Smoothie Vegetarian

STRAWBERRY GREEN GODDESS SMOOTHIE

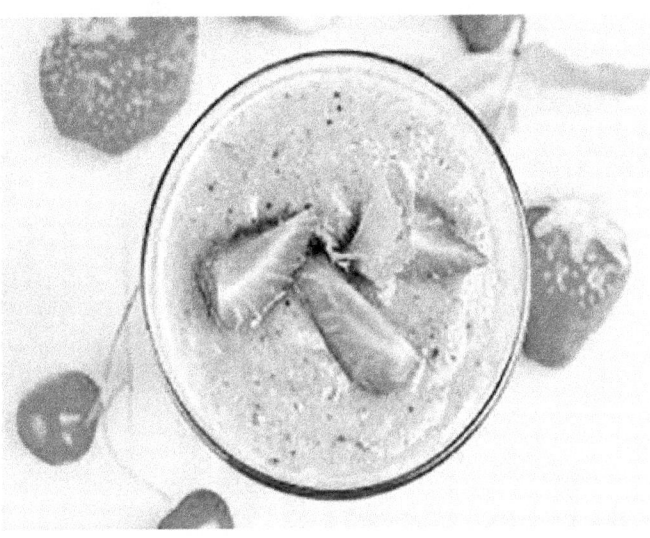

Ingredients

- » 160g ripe strawberries, hulled
- » 160g baby spinach
- » 1 small avocado, halved and the flesh scooped out
- » 150ml pot bio yogurt
- » 2 small oranges, juiced, plus ½ tsp finely grated zest

Preparation

- » Put all the ingredients in a blender and whizz until completely smooth. If it's a little thick, add a drop of chilled water then blitz again. Pour into glasses and drink straight away.

GREEN SMOOTHIE

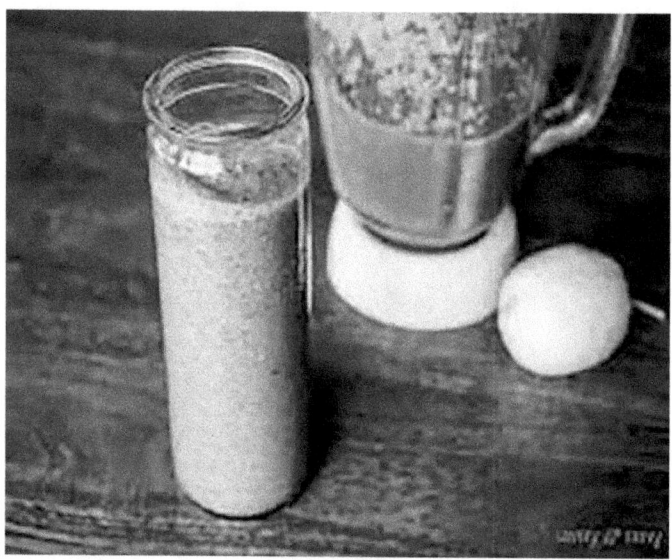

Ingredients

- 1 handful spinach
- (about 50g/2oz), roughly chopped
- 100g broccoli
- florets, roughly chopped
- 2 celery sticks
- 4 tbsp desiccated coconut
- 1 banana
- 300ml rice milk (good dairy alternative - we used one from Rude Health)
- ¼ tsp spirulina or 1 scoop of greens powder or vegan protein powder (optional)

Preparation

» Whizz 300ml water and the ingredients in a blender until smooth.

Avocado Smoothie

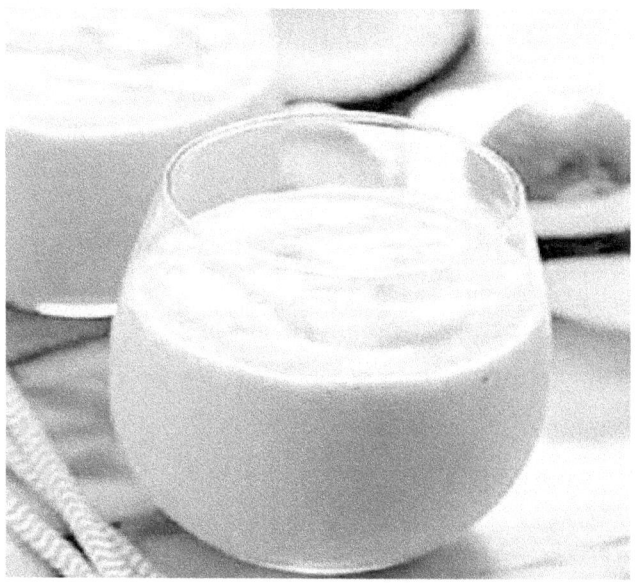

Ingredients

- ½ avocado, peeled, stoned and roughly chopped
- generous handful spinach
- generous handful kale, washed well
- 50g pineapple chunks
- 10cm piece cucumber, roughly chopped
- 300ml coconut water

Preparation

- Put the avocado, spinach, kale, pineapple and cucumber in the blender.
- Top up with coconut water, then blitz until smooth

Carrot and Orange Smoothie

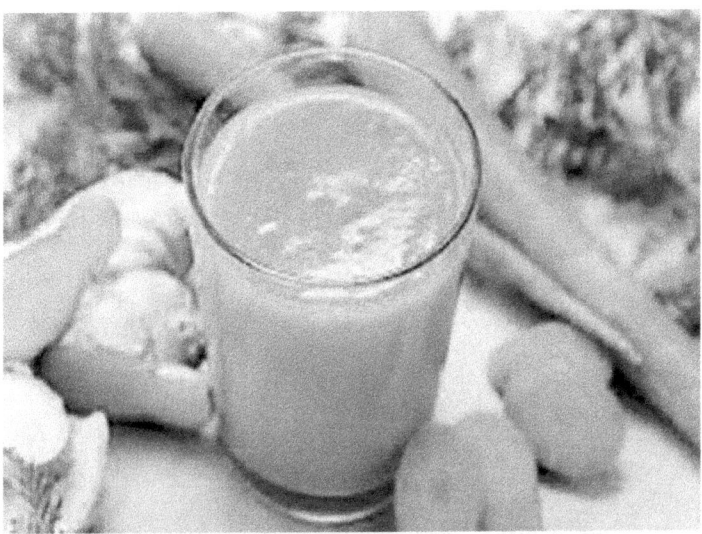

Ingredients

- 2 medium carrots, peeled and roughly chopped or grated depending on your blender
- 2 oranges, peeled
- 2cm piece of ginger, grated
- 2 tbsp oats
- 100g ice

Preparation

- Tip all the ingredients into a blender or smoothie maker and blitz until smooth, adding 150ml water if it's too thick – alter the consistency to your liking.

SUNSHINE SMOOTHIE

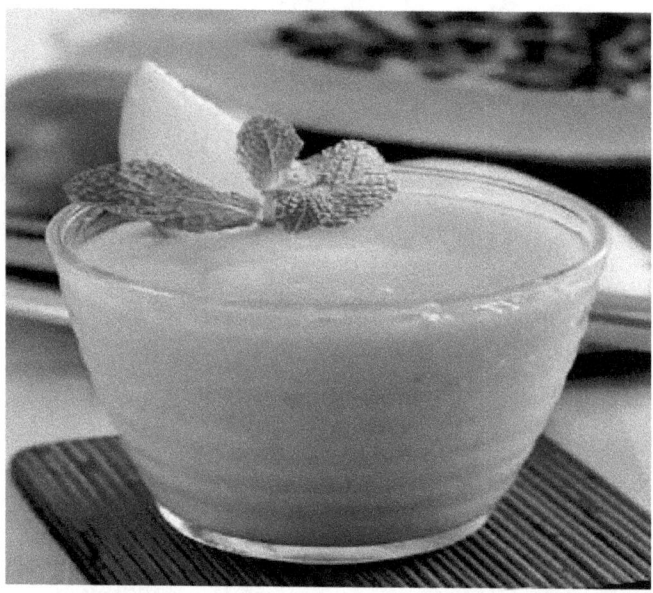

Ingredients

- 500ml carrot juice, chilled
- 200g pineapple (fresh or canned)
- 2 bananas, broken into chunks
- small piece ginger, peeled
- 20g cashew nuts
- juice 1 lime

Preparation

- Put the ingredients in a blender and whizz until smooth. Drink straight away or pour into a bottle to drink on the go. Will keep in the fridge for a day.

Kale smoothie

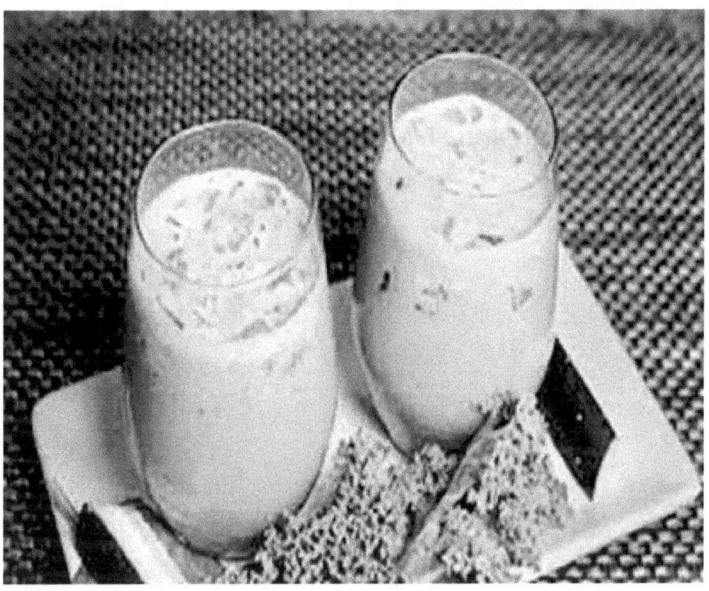

Ingredients

- 2 handfuls kale
- ½ avocado
- ½ lime
- , juice only
- large handful frozen pineapple chunks
- medium-sized chunk ginger
- 1 tbsp cashew nuts
- 1 banana optional

Preparation

» Put all of the ingredients into a bullet or smoothie maker, add a large splash of water and blitz. Add more water until you have the desired consistency.

www.ingramcontent.com/pod-product-compliance
Lightning Source LLC
Chambersburg PA
CBHW080631170426
43209CB00008B/1546